POCKET HANDBOOK
OF PARTICULARLY
EFFECTIVE ACUPOINTS FOR
COMMON CONDITIONS
ILLUSTRATED IN COLOR

of related interest

Pocket Handbook of Body Reflex Zones Illustrated in Color
Guo Changqing Guoyan and Zhaiwei Liu Naigang
ISBN 978 1 84819 119 8
eISBN 978 0 85701 095 7

Pocket Handbook of Particularly Effective Acupoints for Common Conditions Illustrated in Color

GUO CHANGQING GUOYAN
ZHAIWEI LIU NAIGANG

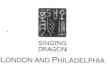

SINGING
DRAGON
LONDON AND PHILADELPHIA

Contributors: Cherui Taolin, Liangchuxi Duanlianhua, Zhongdingwen Zhanghuifang, Wuyuling Feifei, Renqiulan

First edition published in 2010 by People's Military Medical Press

This edition published in 2013
by Singing Dragon
an imprint of Jessica Kingsley Publishers
116 Pentonville Road
London N1 9JB, UK
and
400 Market Street, Suite 400
Philadelphia, PA 19106, USA

www.singingdragon.com

Library of Congress Cataloging in Publication Data
A CIP catalog record for this book is available from the Library of Congress

British Library Cataloguing in Publication Data
A CIP catalogue record for this book is available from the British Library

ISBN 978 1 84819 120 4
eISBN 978 0 85701 094 0

Printed and bound in China

CONTENTS

ABOUT THE BOOK

The book was compiled and edited by senior
specialists and professors of the School of
Acupuncture, Moxibustion and Massage of
Beijing University of Traditional Chinese
Medicine. It outlines key acupuncture points
that are particularly effective in the treatment of
certain conditions and gives standard locations
and indications for the points, along with
providing point names in both Chinese and
English. With clear illustrations, this book assists
readers to locate points precisely. The book is a
useful reference for both teachers and students
of TCM colleges and universities, and clinical
practitioners throughout the world.

Acupuncture therapy is based on the understanding and use of acupuncture points; the therapeutic effect is obtained by stimulation of the points. Therefore, the study of acupuncture points plays an important and central role in the study of acupuncture. Among the numerous acupuncture points, specific points are of utmost importance. Specific acupuncture points are located on the 14 meridians and embody special therapeutic effects and titles; these include five shu points, yuan-source points, luo-connecting points, xi-cleft points, back-shu points, front-mu points, lower he-sea points of the six fu organs, eight influence points, and confluence points of the eight extraordinary vessels.

Specific acupuncture points have gained greater importance through experience in clinical treatment, demonstrating more specific and effective curative capabilities than other less commonly used points. Therefore, to be familiar with and master the usage of these specific acupuncture points is a necessary basis for the study and effective application of acupuncture therapy, as well as being essential for achieving satisfactory improvements in the patient's symptoms.

The book is intended mainly to introduce standard locations and indications of the key specific acupuncture points. It provides illustrations to assist readers in the convenient location and clinical application of acupuncture points. We hope that the publication of this book may add to the collective knowledge and effective use of acupuncture therapy.

CHAPTER 1

Five Shu Antique Points

Section I: Lung Channel of Hand Taiyin; LU

1 少商 (Shàoshāng) LU 11
Lesser Merchant 井穴 Jing-well point of the lung channel

Location: On the radial side of the thumb, 0.1 cun proximal and lateral to the corner of the nail.

Acupuncture:

1. Insert the needle subcutaneously to a depth of 0.1–0.2 cun and stimulate until there is a distending sensation in the local area.

2. Prick with three-edged needle and press tightly to expel 5–13 drops of blood.

Moxibustion: Apply 1–3 moxa cones or hold a moxa stick above the point for 5–10 minutes.

Functions:

- Revives consciousness
- Clears heat and relieves sore throat
- Relieves the surface and clears heat

Indications: Cough, asthma, sore throat, epistaxis and chest distention. Coma, loss of consciousness, epilepsy and infantile convulsions. Vomiting and fever. Spasmodic pain in the thumb and the wrist.

2 鱼际 (Yújì) LU 10 Fish Border 荥穴 Ying-spring point of the lung channel

Location: In the depression proximal to the metacarpophalangeal joint, on the radial side of the midpoint of the metacarpal bone, where the skin changes texture.

Acupuncture:

1. Insert the needle perpendicularly to a depth of 0.3–0.5 cun and stimulate until there is a distending sensation in the local area which radiates to the thumb.

2. Prick with a three-edged needle to bleed.

Moxibustion: Apply 3–5 moxa cones or hold a moxa stick above the point for 3–5 minutes.

Functions:

- Descends lung qi and relieves sore throat
- Clears lung heat and descends rebellious qi
- Harmonizes the stomach and heart

Indications: Hemoptysis, loss of voice, sore throat, dry throat and asthma.

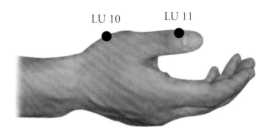

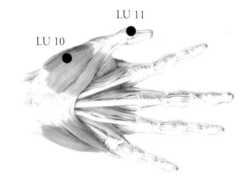

FIGURE 1.1

3 太渊 (Tàiyuān) LU 9 Supreme Abyss 输穴 Shu-stream point of the lung channel

Location: On the transverse wrist crease, on the radial side of the radial artery where the radial pulse is palpable.

Acupuncture:

1. Insert the needle perpendicularly to a depth of 0.2–0.3 cun and stimulate until there is a numb and distending sensation in the local area.

2. Avoid puncturing the radial artery.

Moxibustion:

1. Apply 1–3 moxa cones or hold a moxa stick above the point for 5–10 minutes.

2. Scarring moxibustion is not applicable since the radial artery is located nearby.

Functions:

- Alleviates cough and transforms phlegm
- Descends lung qi
- Regulates and harmonizes the vessels
- Activates the channels and alleviates pain

- Tonifies qi and invigorates the spleen

Indications: Pain in the wrist and pulseless disease (Takayasu's arteritis).

4 经渠 (Jīngqú) LU 8 Channel Gutter 经穴 Jing-river point of the lung channel

Location: On the radial side of the palmar surface of the forearm, 1 cun proximal to the transverse crease of the wrist, in the depression between the styloid process of the radius and the radial artery.

Acupuncture:

1. Insert the needle perpendicularly to a depth of 0.1–0.3 cun and stimulate until there is a sore and numb sensation in the local area radiating to the upper arm.

2. Avoid puncturing the radial artery.

Moxibustion: Apply 3–5 moxa cones, needle-warming moxibustion or, alternatively, hold a moxa stick above the point for 5–10 minutes.

Functions:

- Descends lung qi and alleviates cough and wheezing
- Regulates qi in the chest

Indications: Cough, asthma, hemoptysis, loss of voice, chest congestion and cardiac pain. Headache, tooth ache, pain in the wrist and pulseless disease (Takayasu's arteritis).

5 尺泽 (Chǐzé) LU 5 Cubital Marsh
合穴 He-sea point of lung channel

Location: On the transverse cubital crease, at the radial side of the tendon of muscle biceps brachii.

Acupuncture:

1. Insert the needle perpendicularly to a depth of 0.5–0.8 cun and stimulate until there is a sore and numb sensation in the local area with an electric sensation radiating to the forearm and palm.
2. Prick with a three-edged needle to bleed.

Moxibustion: Apply 7 moxa cones, needle-warming moxibustion or, alternatively, hold a moxa stick above the point for 10 minutes.

Functions:

- Nourishes yin and moisturizes the lung
- Clears heat of the lung
- Descends rebellious qi and alleviates cough
- Regulates the fluid passage way
- Activates the channels, relaxes the sinews and alleviates pain

Indications: Cough, asthma, hemoptysis, sore throat and chest distention. Infantile convulsions. Vomiting and diarrhea. Spasmodic pain of the elbow and arm. Fever.

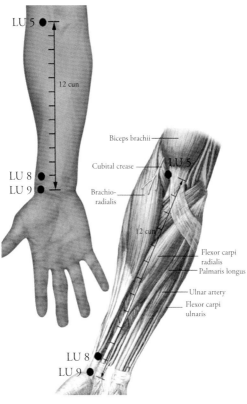

LU 5

12 cun

LU 8
LU 9

Biceps brachii
Cubital crease
LU 5
Brachio-
radialis
12 cun
Flexor carpi
radialis
Palmaris longus
Ulnar artery
Flexor carpi
ulnaris

LU 8
LU 9

FIGURE 1.2

Section II: Heart Channel of Hand Shaoyin; HT

1 少冲 (Shàochōng) HT 9
Lesser Rushing 井穴 Jing-well point of the heart channel

Location: On the radial side of the distal aspect of the little finger, 0.1 cun proximal and lateral to the radial corner of the nail.

Acupuncture:

1. Insert the needle to a depth of 0.1–0.2 cun and stimulate until there is a sore and distending sensation in the local area.

2. Prick with a three-edged needle to bleed.

Moxibustion: Apply 3–5 moxa cones or hold a moxa stick above the point for 5–10 minutes.

Functions:

- Revives consciousness
- Clears heat and calms the spirit
- Benefits the throat, tongue and eyes

Indications: Cardiac pain, heart palpitation and chest pain. Epilepsy, stroke and loss of consciousness. Fever.

2 少府 (Shàofǔ) HT 8 Small Mansion 荥穴 Ying-spring point of the heart channel

Location: In the palm, between the 4th and 5th metacarpal bones. When the hand makes a loose fist the point is located under the tip of the little finger.

Acupuncture: Insert the needle perpendicularly to a depth of 0.3–0.5 cun and stimulate until the needling sensation radiates to the elbow or the little finger.

Moxibustion: Apply 3–5 moxa cones or hold a moxa stick above the point for 5–7 minutes.

Functions:

- Clears heat in the heart and small intestine
- Calms the spirit
- Activates the channels and alleviates pain

Indications: Heart palpitations and chest pain.

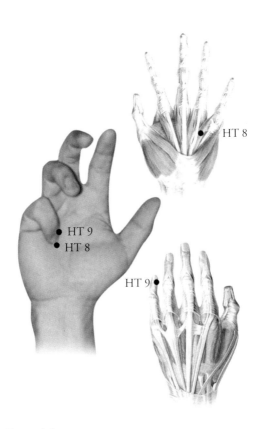

FIGURE 1.3

3 神門 (Shénmén) HT 7
Spirit Door 輸穴 Shu-stream point of the heart channel

Location: On the transverse crease of the wrist on the radial side of the tendon of the muscle flexor carpi ulnaris.

Acupuncture:

1. Insert the needle perpendicularly to a depth of 0.3–0.5 cun and stimulate until there is soreness and numbness in the local area with an electrical sensation radiating to the fingers.

2. Insert the needle obliquely towards HT 4 (lingdào) to a depth of 1.0–1.5 cun and stimulate until there is a sore and numb sensation in the local area radiating to the upper arm.

Moxibustion: Apply 1–3 moxa cones or hold a moxa stick above the point for 5–15 minutes.

Functions:

- Clears heat and calms the spirit
- Regulates and tonifies the heart

Indications: Irritability, amnesia, insomnia, loss of consciousness and epilepsy. Cardiac pain and palpitations.

4 灵道 (Língdào) HT 4 Spirit Path 经穴 Jing-river point of the heart channel

Location: On the medial aspect of the forearm, on the line connecting HT 7 (shénmén) to HT 3 (shàohǎi), 1.5 cun proximal to HT 7 (shénmén).

Acupuncture: Insert the needle perpendicularly to a depth of 0.5–0.8 cun and stimulate until there is a sore, numb sensation in the local area radiating to the elbow and fingers.

Moxibustion: Apply 1–3 moxa cones or hold a moxa stick above the point for 10–20 minutes.

Functions:

- Calms the spirit
- Relaxes the muscles and sinews

Indications: Heart palpitations, terrors and cardiac pain.

5 少海 (Shàohǎi) HT 3 Lesser Sea 合穴 He-sea point of the heart channel

Location: At the midpoint of the line connecting the medial end of the transverse crease of the elbow to the medial epicondyle of the humerus when the elbow is flexed.

Acupuncture: Insert the needle perpendicularly to a depth of 0.5–1.0 cun and stimulate until there is a sore, numbness in the local area or an electric sensation radiating to the forearm.

Moxibustion: Apply 3–5 moxa cones or needle-warming moxibustion or, alternatively, hold a moxa stick above the point for 5–10 minutes.

Functions:

- Clears heat and calms the spirit
- Activates the channels and regulates qi

Indications: Cardiac pain. Spasmodic pain and numbness of the elbow and arm. Sudden loss of voice.

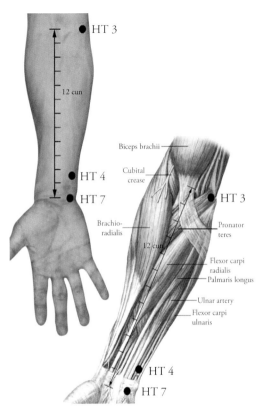

HT 3

12 cun

HT 4
HT 7

Biceps brachii

Cubital
crease

HT 3

Brachio-
radialis

Pronator
teres

12 cun

Flexor carpi
radialis
Palmaris longus

Ulnar artery

Flexor carpi
ulnaris

HT 4
HT 7

FIGURE 1.4

Section III: Pericardium Channel of Hand Jueyin; PC

1 中冲 (Zhōngchōng) PC 9 Central Rushing 井穴 Jing-well point of the pericardium channel

Location: In the center of the tip of the distal phalanx of the middle finger.

Acupuncture:

1. Insert the needle to a depth of 0.1–0.2 cun and stimulate until there is a sore and distending sensation in the local area.

2. Prick with a three-edged needle to bleed.

Moxibustion: Apply 1–3 moxa cones or hold a moxa stick above the point for 5–10 minutes.

Functions:

- Clears heat from the pericardium and revives consciousness
- Clears summer heat and cools the blood

Indications: Cardiac pain and irritability. Stroke, febrile diseases without sweating and heatstroke. Redness of eyes or tongue and infantile night crying.

2 劳宫 (Láogōng) PC 8 Palace of Labour 荥穴 Ying-spring point of the pericardium channel

Location: In the center of the palm, between the 2nd and 3rd metacarpal bones, closer to the 3rd metacarpal bone. When a loose fist is made, the point lies under the tip of the 3rd finger.

Acupuncture: Insert the needle perpendicularly to a depth of 0.3–0.5 cun and stimulate until there is a sore, numb sensation in the local area radiating to the palm.

Moxibustion: Apply moxa cones or hold a moxa stick above the point for 3–5 minutes.

Functions:

- Clears heart heat and cools the blood
- Calms the spirit
- Tonifies stomach yin
- Clears heat of the middle jiao
- Revives consciousness

Indications: Hyperactivity, epilepsy and child-hood convulsions. Irritability and halitosis.

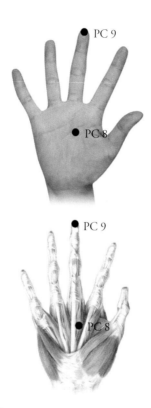

FIGURE 1.5

3 大陵 (Dàlíng) PC 7 Great Mound 输穴 Shu-stream point of the pericardium channel

Location: On the palmar aspect of the forearm, in the center of the transverse crease of the wrist.

Acupuncture:

1. Insert the needle perpendicularly to a depth of 0.3–0.5 cun and stimulate until there is a sore, numb sensation in the local area with an electric sensation radiating to the finger tip.

2. Insert the needle perpendicularly into the wrist and stimulate until there is a sore and numb sensation in the local area.

3. Prick with a three-edged needle to bleed.

Moxibustion: Apply 3–5 moxa cones or hold a moxa stick above the point for 10–20 minutes.

Functions:

- Descends rebellious qi and regulates the stomach
- Clears heart heat and calms the spirit
- Unbinds the chest and regulates qi

- Activates the channels and cools blood

Indications: Cardiac pain, palpitations and irritability.

4 间使 (Jiānshǐ) PC 5 Intermediary Courier 经穴 Jing-river point of the pericardium channel

Location: On the palmar aspect of the forearm, 3 cun superior to the transverse crease of the wrist, on the line connecting PC 3 (qū zé) to PC 7 (dà ling).

Acupuncture: Insert the needle perpendicularly towards TH 6 (zhī gōu) to a depth of 0.5–0.8 cun and stimulate until there is a sore, numbness in the local area with an electric shock sensation radiating to the finger.

Moxibustion: Apply 3–5 moxa cones or hold a moxa stick above the point for 5–10 minutes.

Functions:
- Unbinds the chest and transforms phlegm
- Calms the spirit

- Descends rebellious qi and regulates the stomach
- Regulates menstruation

Indications: Malaria.

5 曲泽 (Qūzé) PC 3 Crooked Marsh 合穴 He-sea point of the pericardium channel

Location: On the transverse crease of the elbow, on the ulnar side of the tendon of muscle biceps brachii.

Acupuncture:

1. Insert the needle perpendicularly to a depth of 0.5–1.0 cun and stimulate until there is a numb, distending sensation in the local area radiating to the middle finger.
2. Prick with a three-edged needle to bleed.
3. Avoid puncturing the vessel.

Moxibustion: Apply 3–5 moxa cones or hold a moxa stick above the point for 5–10 minutes.

Functions:

- Clears summer heat
- Harmonizes the stomach and stops vomiting
- Tonifies heart qi
- Activates the channels and alleviates pain

Indications: Dryness of the mouth, vomiting and hematemesis. Spasms and pain in the elbow and arm. Cholera and measles.

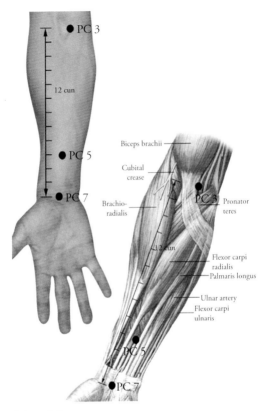

FIGURE 1.6

Section IV: Large Intestine Channel of Hand Yangming; LI

1 商阳 (Shāngyáng) LI 1 Merchant Yang 井穴 Jing-well point of the large intestine channel

Location: On the radial side of the index finger, 0.1 cun proximal and medial to the corner of the nail.

Acupuncture:

1. Insert the needle perpendicularly to a depth of 0.1–0.2 cun and stimulate until there is a distending sensation in the local area.

2. Prick with a three-edged needle to bleed.

Moxibustion: Apply 1–3 moxa cones or hold a moxa stick above the point for 5–10 minutes.

Functions:

- Relieves the surface and clears heat
- Relieves sore throat and alleviates pain
- Revives consciousness

Indications: Sore throat, dryness of the mouth, tooth ache, deafness and tinnitus. Fainting and stroke. Fever and febrile diseases with anhidrosis.

2 二间 (Erjiān) LI 2 Second Interval 荥穴 Ying-spring point of the large intestine channel

Location: On the radial side of the index finger, when a loose fist is made the point is in the depression distal to the metacarpalphalangeal joint, at the junction where the skin changes texture.

Acupuncture: Insert the needle perpendicularly to a depth of 0.2–0.4 cun and stimulate until there is a distending sensation in the local area.

Moxibustion: Apply 3–5 moxa cones or hold a moxa stick above the point for 5–10 minutes.

Functions:

- Relieves the surface and clears heat
- Relieves sore throat
- Expels wind and clears heat
- Activates the channel and alleviates pain

Indications: Tooth ache, dryness of the mouth and facial paralysis.

3 三间 (Sānjiān) LI 3 Third Interval 输穴 Shu-stream point of the large intestine channel

Location: On the radial side of the index finger, when a loose fist is made the point is in the depression proximal to the head of the 2nd metacarpal bone.

Acupuncture: Insert the needle perpendicularly to a depth of 0.3–0.5 cun and stimulate until there is a numb, distending sensation in the local area radiating to the dorsum of hand.

Moxibustion: Apply 3–5 moxa cones or needle-warming moxibustion or alternatively hold a moxa stick above the point for 5–10 minutes.

Functions:

- Expels wind and clears heat
- Benefits the throat and teeth
- Dispels fullness and treats diarrhea
- Regulates qi of the large intestine

Indications: Tooth ache, sore throat and fever.

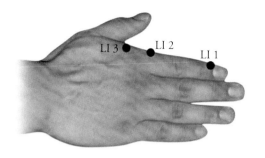

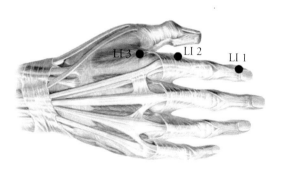

FIGURE 1.7

4 阳溪 (Yángxī) LI 5 Yang Stream 经穴 Jing-river point of the large intestine channel

Location: On the dorsal side of the wrist, in the depression between the tendons of muscles extensor pollicis longus and extensor pollicis brevis.

Acupuncture: Insert the needle perpendicularly to a depth of 0.5–0.8 cun and stimulate until there is a sore, numb sensation in the local area.

Moxibustion: Apply 3–5 moxa cones or needle-warming moxibustion or, alternatively, hold a moxa stick above the point for 10–20 minutes.

Functions:

- Expels wind and clears heat
- Reduces swelling and alleviates pain
- Clears yangming fire
- Benefits the wrist joint

Indications: Headache, redness, swelling and pain in the eyes, deafness, tinnitus and sore throat. Pain in the wrist.

5 曲池 (Qǔchí) LI 11 Crooked Pond 合穴 He-sea point of the large intestine channel

Location: In the depression at the radial end of the transverse cubital crease when the elbow is flexed.

Acupuncture:

1. Insert the needle perpendicularly to a depth of 1.0–1.5 cun and stimulate until there is a sore, numb sensation in the local area radiating to either the shoulder or the fingers.

2. Insert the needle deeply in the direction of HT 3 (shàohǎi) and stimulate until there is a sore, numb sensation in the local area radiating to the shoulder or the fingers.

3. Apply the "Hegu Puncture" or "Triple Puncture" technique.

4. Insert the needle obliquely towards the elbow and stimulate until there is a radiating sensation speading to the fingers.

5. Prick with a three-edged needle to bleed.

Moxibustion: Apply 5–7 moxa cones or needle-warming moxibustion or, alternatively, hold a moxa stick above the point for 5–20 minutes.

Functions:

- Clears heat and cools blood
- Drains dampness
- Expels wind and alleviates itching
- Regulates qi and blood
- Activates collaterals to relieve pain

Indications: Swelling and pain in the throat, coughing and asthma. Abdominal pain, vomiting, diarrhea, dysentery constipation and intestinal carbuncles. Tooth ache, pain and redness of the eyes and blurred vision. Itrismus epilepsy and high blood pressure. Measles, sores, scabies, exanthemata and erysipelas. Redness and swelling of the arms, paralysis of the upper limbs, pain and paralysis of the elbow and shoulder. Fever.

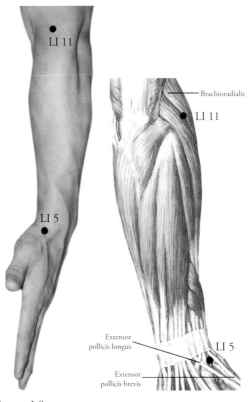

LI 11

Brachioradialis

LI 11

LI 5

Extensor
pollicis longus

Extensor
pollicis brevis

LI 5

FIGURE 1.8

Section V: Small Intestine Channel of Hand Taiyang; SI

1 少泽 (Shàozé) SI 1 Lesser Marsh 井穴 Jing-well point of the small intestine channel

Location: On the ulnar side of the distal phalanx of the little finger, 0.1 cun proximal and lateral to the corner of the nail.

Acupuncture:

1. Insert the needle to a depth of 0.1–0.2 cun and stimulate until there is a distending, painful sensation in the local area.

2. Prick with a three-edged needle to bleed.

Moxibustion: Apply 1–3 moxa cones or hold a moxa stick above the point for 5–10 minutes.

Functions:

- Clears heat
- Revives consciousness
- Promotes lactation and benefits the breasts

Indications: Stroke. Headache, deafness, sore throat and stiffness of the tongue. Insufficient lactation. Febrile disease.

2 前谷 (Qiángǔ) SI 2 Anterior Valley 荥穴 Ying-spring point of the small intestine channel

Location: On the ulnar side of the hand, distal to the 5th metacarpophalangeal joint, at the end of the transverse crease, at the junction where the skin changes texture.

Acupuncture: Insert the needle perpendicularly to a depth of 0.2–0.3 cun and stimulate until there is a sore, distending sensation in the local area.

Moxibustion: Apply 1–3 moxa cones or hold a moxa stick above the point for 5–10 minutes.

Functions:

- Relieves superficial excess by promoting cooling
- Revives consciousness
- Benefits the eyes, ears, nose and throat
- Activates the channels and alleviates pain

Indications: Eye pain, lacrimation, tinnitus, epistaxis, cheek pain and sore throat. Pain and rigidity of the head and neck, neck stiffness and arm pain.

3 后溪 (Hòuxī) SI 3 Posterior Valley 输穴 Shu-stream point of the small intestine channel

Location: On the ulnar side of the hand, proximal to the 5th metacarpophalangeal joint, at the end of the transverse crease, at the junction where the skin changes texture.

Acupuncture: Insert the needle perpendicularly to a depth of 0.5–0.8 cun and stimulate until there is a sore, numb sensation in the local area spreading to the palm.

Moxibustion: Apply 1–3 moxa cones or hold a moxa stick above the point for 5–10 minutes.

Functions:

- Activates the channel and alleviates pain
- Clears wind and heat
- Calms the spirit and treats epilepsy
- Regulates the governing vessel
- Benefits the occiput, neck and back
- Revives consciousness

Indications: Tinnitus and deafness. Manic psychosis, epilepsy and stroke. Pain and rigidity of the head and neck. Febrile conditions, jaundice and malaria.

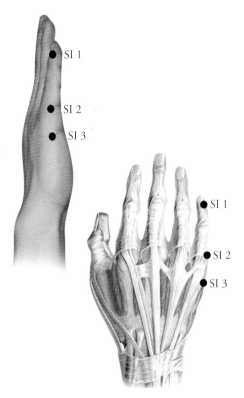

FIGURE 1.9

4 阳谷 (Yánggǔ) SI 5 Yang Valley 经穴 Jing-river point of the small intestine channel

Location: On the ulnar side of the wrist, in the depression between the styloid process of the ulna and the pisiform bone.

Acupuncture: Insert the needle perpendicularly to a depth of 0.3–0.5 cun and stimulate until there is a sore, numb sensation in the local area radiating to the wrist.

Moxibustion: Apply 3–5 moxa cones or needle-warming moxibustion or, alternatively, hold a moxa stick above the point for 5–10 minutes.

Functions:

- Clears heat and calms the spirit
- Benefits the ears and eyes

Indications: Disorders of the head and five sense organs: headache, tinnitus, deafness and eye pain. Disorders manifesting along the small intestine channel: pain and weakness of the shoulder.

5 小海 (Xiǎohǎi) SI 8 Small Sea 合穴 He-sea point of the small intestine channel

Location: On the medial aspect of the elbow, in the depression between the olecranon and the medial epicondyle of the humerus.

Acupuncture: Insert the needle perpendicularly to a depth of 0.2–0.3 cun and stimulate until there is a sore, numb sensation in the local area or until there is an electric shock sensation down the ulnar aspect of the forearm and hand.

Moxibustion: Apply 3–5 moxa cones or needle-warming moxibustion or, alternatively, hold a moxa stick above the point for 5–10 minutes.

Functions:

- Clears heat and calms the spirit
- Activates the channel and alleviates pain
- Regulates qi and blood

Indications: Disorders of the head and five sense organs: headache, deafness, blurred vision and swelling of the gums. Manic psychosis and epilepsy.

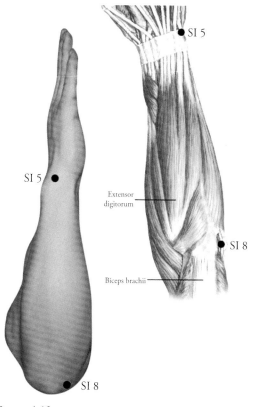

Extensor
digitorum

Biceps brachii

FIGURE 1.10

Section VI: Three Heater Channel of Hand Shaoyang; TH

1 关冲 (Guānchōng) TH 1 Gate Rushing 井穴 Jing-well point of the three heater channel

Location: On the ulnar aspect of the distal phalanx of the ring finger, 0.1 cun proximal and lateral to the ulnar side of the corner of the nail on the ring finger.

Acupuncture:

1. Insert the needle perpendicularly to a depth of 0.1–0.3 cun and stimulate until there is a sore, distending sensation in the local area radiating to the palm.

2. Prick with a three-edged needle to bleed.

Moxibustion: Apply 3–5 moxa cones or hold a moxa stick above the point for 5–10 minutes.

Functions:

- Expels wind and clears heat
- Activates the channel and alleviates pain
- Revives consciousness

Indications: Headache, dizziness, redness of the eyes, deafness, tinnitus and sore throat. Febrile diseases without sweating.

2 液门 (Yèmén) TH 2 Door of Fluids 荥穴 Ying-spring point of the three heater channel

Location: On the dorsum aspect of the hand, proximal to the margin of the web between the 4th and 5th finger, at the junction where the skin changes texture.

Acupuncture:

1. Insert the needle perpendicularly to a depth of 0.3–0.5 cun and stimulate until there is a sore and distending sensation in the local area radiating to the dorsum of the hand.

2. Insert the needle obliquely upwards towards the wrist and stimulate until there is a sensation in the local area radiating to the elbow and along the channel.

Moxibustion: Apply 3–5 moxa cones or hold a moxa stick above the point for 5–10 minutes.

Functions:

- Clears heat and calms the spirit
- Activates channel and alleviates pain

Indications: Headache, dizziness, redness of the eyes, deafness, tinnitus. Febrile diseases without sweating. Malaria.

3 中渚 (Zhōngzhǔ) TH 3 输穴
Shu-stream point of the
three heater channel

Location: On the dorsum aspect of the hand, proximal to the 4th metacarpophalangeal joint, in the depression between the 4th and 5th metacarpal bones.

Acupuncture:

1. Insert the needle perpendicularly to a depth of 0.3–0.5 cun and stimulate until there is a sore, distending sensation in the local area with an electric sensation radiating to the tip of the finger.

2. Insert the needle obliquely to a depth of 0.5–1.0 cun and stimulate until there is a sore, numb sensation in the local area radiating to the wrist.

Moxibustion: Apply 3–5 moxa cones or needle-warming moxibustion or, alternatively, hold a moxa stick above the point for 5–10 minutes.

Functions:

- Expels wind and clears heat
- Activates the channel and alleviates pain
- Benefits the eyes and ears

Indications: Headache, redness and pain in the eyes, deafness, tinnitus and sore throat. An inability to flex and extend the fingers.

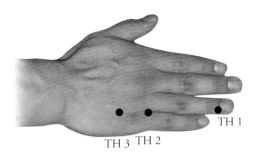

TH 3   TH 2

TH 1

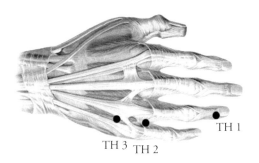

TH 3   TH 2

TH 1

FIGURE 1.11

4 支沟 (Zhīgōu) TH 6 Branch Ditch 经穴 Jing-river point of the three heater channel

Location: On the dorsal aspect of the forearm, on the line between TH 4 (yang chí) and the olecranon, 3 cun above the transverse crease of the wrist, between the ulna and radius.

Acupuncture:

1. Insert the needle perpendicularly to a depth of 0.5–1.0 cun and stimulate until there is a sore, numb sensation in the local area radiating to the elbow and sometimes with an electric sensation radiating to the tip of the finger.

2. Insert the needle obliquely to a depth of 1.5–2.0 cun and stimulate until there is a sore, numb sensation in the local area radiating to the elbow and shoulder.

Moxibustion: Apply 3–5 moxa cones or needle-warming moxibustion or, alternatively, hold a moxa stick above the point for 10–20 minutes.

Functions:

- Regulates qi and clears heat

- Relieves congestion in the chest and descends rebellious qi
- Activates the channel and alleviates pain
- Benefits the uterus

Indications: Chest and hypochondriac pain. Constipation.

5 天井 (Tiānjǐng) TH 10
Heavenly Well 合穴 He-sea point
of the three heater channel

Location: On the posterior aspect of the arm when the elbow is flexed, in the depression 1 cun proximal to the tip of the elbow.

Acupuncture: Insert the needle perpendicularly to a depth of 0.5–1.0 cun and stimulate until there is a sore, numb sensation in the local area.

Moxibustion: Apply 3–5 moxa cones or needle-warming moxibustion or, alternatively, hold a moxa stick above the point for 10–20 minutes.

Functions:

- Regulates qi and transforms phlegm
- Relieves congestion in the chest and descends rebellious qi
- Clears heat and calms the spirit
- Activates the channel and alleviates pain

Indications: Sudden loss of voice, deafness, tooth ache and eye conditions. Pain in the arm.

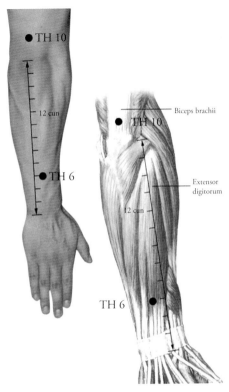

FIGURE 1.12

Section VII: Stomach Channel of Foot Yangming; ST

1 厉兑 (Lìduì) ST 45 井穴 Jing-well point of the stomach channel

Location: On the lateral aspect of the 2nd toe, 0.1 cun proximal and lateral to the corner of the nail.

Acupuncture:

1. Insert the needle to a depth of 0.1–0.2 cun and stimulate until there is a sore, distending sensation in the local area.
2. Prick with three-edged needle to bleed.

Moxibustion: Apply 1–3 moxa cones or hold a moxa stick above the point for 5–10 minutes.

Functions:

- Clears heat of the stomach channel
- Calms the spirit and restores consciousness
- Dredges the course of the channel

Indications: Insomnia with copious dreams.

2 内庭 (Nèitíng) ST 44 Inner Courtyard 荥穴 Ying-spring point of the stomach channel

Location: On the dorsum of foot, distal to the 2nd metatarsophalangeal joint, in the web between the 2nd and 3rd toes.

Acupuncture:

1. Insert the needle perpendicularly or obliquely to a depth of 0.3–0.5 cun and stimulate until there is a sore, numb sensation in the local area.

2. Insert the needle obliquely upwards and stimulate until the sensation radiates to the tibia, abdomen, stomach and face.

Moxibustion: Apply 3–5 moxa cones or hold a moxa stick above the point for 5–10 minutes.

Functions:

- Clears fire in the stomach channel and alleviates pain

- Harmonizes the intestines and clears damp-heat
- Regulates the yangming channels

Indications: Abdominal pain and distention, diarrhea and dysentery. Tooth ache, sore throat and epistaxis. Irritability, insomnia with copious dreams and psychosis.

3 陷谷 (Xiàngǔ) ST 43 Sinking Valley 输穴 Shu-stream point of the stomach channel

Location: On the dorsum of the foot, in the depression proximal to the junction of the 2nd and 3rd metatarsophalangeal joint.

Acupuncture:

1. Insert the needle perpendicularly to a depth of 0.3–0.5 cun and stimulate until there is a sore, numb sensation in the local area radiating to the dorsum of the foot.

2. Insert the needle obliquely upward to a depth of 0.5–1.0 cun and stimulate until there is a sore, numb sensation in the local area radiating to the dorsum of the foot.

Moxibustion: Apply 3–5 moxa cones or hold a moxa stick above the point for 5–10 minutes.

Functions:

- Relieves exterior pathogens by promoting cooling
- Invigorates the spleen and dispels edema
- Harmonizes the stomach and intestines

Indications: Borborygmus and abdominal pain.

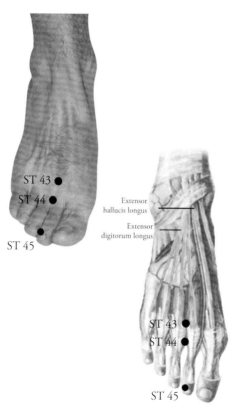

ST 43 ●
ST 44 ●

Extensor
hallucis longus

Extensor
digitorum longus

ST 45 ●

ST 43 ●
ST 44 ●

ST 45 ●

FIGURE 1.13

4 解溪 (Jiěxī) ST 41 Dispersing Stream 经穴 Jing-river point of the stomach channel

Location: On the transverse malleolus crease of the dorsum of the foot, between the tendons of the muscles extensor pollicis longus and extensor digitorum longus.

Acupuncture:

1. Insert the needle perpendicularly to a depth of 0.3–0.5 cun and stimulate until there is a sore, numb sensation in the local area radiating to the ankle.

2. Insert the needle to a depth of 1.0–1.5 cun in the direction of GB 40 (qiū xū) or SP 5 (shāng qiū) and stimulate until there is a sore, numb sensation in the local area spreading in the ankle.

Moxibustion: Apply 3–5 moxa cones or hold a moxa stick above the point for 5–10 minutes.

Functions:

- Clears heat in the stomach and transforms phlegm
- Activates the channel and alleviates pain
- Calms the spirit

Indications: Redness of the eyes and headache. Abdominal distention and constipation. Pain, weakness and numbness of the legs.

5 足三里 (Zúsānlǐ) ST 36 Three Leg Miles 合穴 He-sea point of the stomach channel

Location: On the anterior aspect of the lower leg, 3 cun distal to ST 35 (dúbí), one finger's breadth lateral from the anterior ridge of the tibia.

Acupuncture:

1. Insert the needle perpendicularly to a depth of 0.5–1.5 cun and stimulate until there is a sensation radiating to the ankle and dorsum of the foot and toes.

2. Insert the needle obliquely upwards and stimulate until there is a sensation radiating to ST 31 (bìguān), ST 29 (guīlái) and ST 25 (tiānshū).

Moxibustion: Apply 5–10 moxa cones or needle-warming moxibustion or, alternatively, hold a moxa stick over the point for 10–20 minutes. Apply scarring moxibustion once a year or apply 5–10 moxa cones once a day, 20 days a month, to promote general health and well-being.

Functions:

- Invigorates the spleen and harmonizes the stomach
- Supports correct qi and nourishes original qi
- Activates the channel and alleviates pain
- Regulates qi and resolves dampness

- Tonifies qi and nourishes blood
- Prevents disease and benefits macrobiosis

Indications: Stomach ache, vomiting, abdominal distention, borborygmus, indigestion, diarrhea, constipation and dysentery. Epilepsy and stroke. Wheezing with phlegm, carbuncle weakness and hemoptysis. Dysuria, enuresis and hernia. Palpitations. Gynecological disorders: eclampsia, bloody and excessive leucorrhea, dysmenorrhea and postnatal lumbago. Pain in the knee and shin, paralysis of the lower limbs, sciatica and general conditions of the knee and local area. Irritability, beriberi and insomnia.

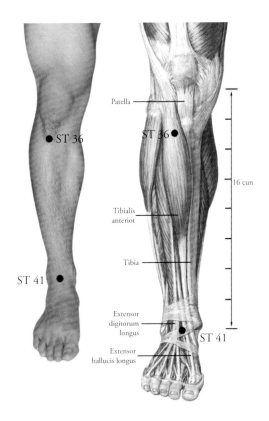

Patella

ST 36

16 cun

Tibialis
anteriot

Tibia

Extensor
digitorum
longus

ST 41

Extensor
hallucis longus

ST 36

ST 41

FIGURE 1.14

Section VIII: Bladder Channel of Foot Taiyang; BL

1 至阴 (Zhìyīn) BL 67 Reaching Yin 井穴 Jing-well point of the bladder channel

Location: On the lateral aspect of the little toe, 0.1 cun proximal and lateral to the corner of the nail.

Acupuncture:

1. Insert the needle perpendicularly to a depth of 0.1–0.2 cun and stimulate until there is a sore, numb sensation in the local area.
2. Prick with a three-edged needle to bleed.

Moxibustion: Apply 3–5 moxa cones or needle-warming moxibustion or, alternatively, hold a moxa stick above the point for 10–20 minutes.

Functions:

- Expels wind and clears the head and eyes
- Turns the foetus and facilitates labour
- Regulates qi and blood

Indications: Headache, nasal obstruction, epistaxis and eye pain. Malposition of the fetus and difficult labor. Hot sensations on the sole of the foot.

2 足通谷 (Zútōnggǔ) BL 66 Valley Passage of the Foot 荥穴 Ying-spring point of the bladder channel

Location: On the lateral aspect of the foot, anterior to the 5th metatarsophalangeal joint, at the junction where the skin changes texture.

Acupuncture: Insert the needle perpendicularly to a depth of 0.3–0.5 cun and stimulate until there is a sore, numb sensation in the local area.

Moxibustion: Apply 3–7 moxa cones or needle-warming moxibustion or, alternatively, hold a moxa stick above the point for 5–10 minutes.

Functions:

- Relaxes sinews, activates the channel and alleviates pain
- Clears the head and benefits mental capacity

Indications: Headache and neck stiffness.

3 束骨 (Shùgǔ) BL 65 Restraining Bone 输穴 Shu-stream point of the bladder channel

Location: On the lateral aspect of the foot, posterior to the 5th metatarsophalangeal joint, at the junction where the skin changes texture.

Acupuncture: Insert the needle perpendicularly to a depth of 0.3–0.5 cun and stimulate until there is a sore, numb sensation in the local area.

Moxibustion: Apply 3–7 moxa cones or needle-warming moxibustion or, alternatively, hold a moxa stick above the point for 5–10 minutes.

Functions:

- Relaxes sinews, activates the channel and alleviates pain
- Clears heat and expels wind

Indications: Headache and pain in the lateral side of the lower extremities.

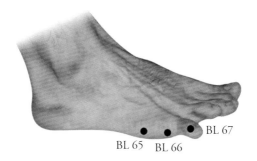

BL 67

BL 65   BL 66

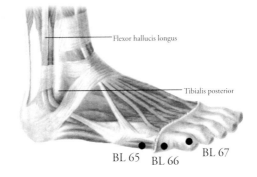

Flexor hallucis longus

Tibialis posterior

BL 65   BL 66   BL 67

FIGURE 1.15

4 昆仑 (Kūnlún) BL 60 Kunlun Mountains 经穴 Jing-river point of the bladder channel

Location: On the foot, posterior to the lateral malleolus, in the depression between the tip of the lateral malleolus and tendon calcaneus.

Acupuncture:

1. Insert the needle perpendicularly towards KI 3 (tàixī) to a depth of 0.5–1.5 cun and stimulate until there is a sore, numb sensation in the local area radiating to the heel.

2. Insert the needle obliquely towards BL 59 (fū yang) to a depth of 2.0–3.0 cun.

Moxibustion: Apply 5–9 moxa cones or needle-warming moxibustion or, alternatively, hold a moxa stick above the point for 10–20 minutes.

Functions:

- Relaxes sinews, activates the channel and alleviates pain
- Regulates the lumbar region and knees

Indications: Headache, dizziness, eye pain and epistaxis. Neck stiffness, lumbosacral pain, spasms and pain in the shoulder, swelling and soreness of the heel.

5 委中 (Wěizhōng) BL 40
Bend Middle 合穴 He-sea
point of the bladder channel

Location: At the midpoint of the transverse popliteal crease in the center of the popliteal fossa, between the tendon of the muscles biceps femoris and semitendinous.

Acupuncture:

1. Insert the needle perpendicularly to a depth of 0.5–1.0 cun and stimulate until there is a sore, distending and numb sensation radiating to the calf and foot.

2. Prick with a three-edged needle to bleed.

Moxibustion: Apply 3–5 moxa cones or needle-warming moxibustion or, alternatively, hold a moxa stick above the point for 10–20 minutes.

Functions:

- Benefits the lumbar region and knees
- Activates the channel and alleviates pain
- Cools blood and clears summer heat
- Stops vomiting and diarrhea

Indications: Lumbar pain, joint pain due to stagnation of damp-cold and hemiplegia. Erysipelas, boils, furuncles, bruises and spontaneous bleeding under the skin. Abdominal pain, vomiting and diarrhea.

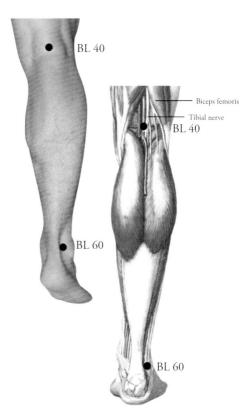

BL 40

Biceps femoris

Tibial nerve

BL 40

BL 60

BL 60

FIGURE 1.16

Section IX: Gallbladder Channel of Foot Shaoyang; GB

1 足窍阴 (Zúqiàoyīn) GB 44 Foot Cavity of Yin 井穴 Jing-well point of the gallbladder channel

Location: On the lateral aspect of the 4th toe, 0.1 cun proximal and lateral to the corner of the nail.

Acupuncture:

1. Insert the needle subcutaneously to a depth of 0.1–0.2 cun and stimulate until there is a sore, numb sensation in the local area.

2. Prick with a three-edged needle to bleed.

Moxibustion: Apply 3–5 moxa cones or needle-warming moxibustion or, alternatively, hold a moxa stick above the point for 5–10 minutes.

Functions:

- Clears heat and pacifies wind
- Calms the spirit and revives consciousness
- Activates the channel and alleviates pain

Indications: Migraine, tinnitus, deafness and eye pain. Pain of the chest and hypochondrium.

2 侠溪 (Xiáxī) GB 43 Narrow Revine 荥穴 Ying-spring point of the gallbladder channel

Location: On the dorsum of the foot, at the margin of the web between the 4th and 5th toes.

Acupuncture: Insert the needle perpendicularly to a depth of 0.5–0.8 cun and stimulate until there is a sore, numb sensation in the local area.

Moxibustion: Apply 3–5 moxa cones or needle-warming moxibustion or, alternatively, hold a moxa stick above the point for 5–10 minutes.

Functions:

- Clears heat and pacifies wind
- Reduces swelling and allevates pain
- Clears dampness and heat in the gallbladder channel

Indications: Headache, tinnitus, deafness and eye pain.

3 足临泣 (Zúlínqì) GB 41 Foot Supervising Tears 输穴 Shu-stream point of the gallbladder channel

Location: On the lateral aspect of the dorsum of the foot, posterior to the 4th metatarsophalangeal joint, in the depression on the lateral aspect of the tendon of the muscle extensor digit minimi of the foot.

Acupuncture:

1. Insert the needle perpendicularly to a depth of 0.5–0.8 cun and stimulate until there is a sore and numb sensation in the local area spreading to the toe.

2. Prick with a three-edged needle to bleed.

Moxibustion: Apply 3–5 moxa cones or needle-warming moxibustion or, alternatively, hold a moxa stick above the point for 5–10 minutes.

Functions:

- Spreads liver qi
- Pacifies wind and clears fire
- Clears the head and benefits the eyes

Indications: Headache, redness, swelling and pain in the eyes, tooth ache and deafness. Dizziness, dyspnea and mastitis.

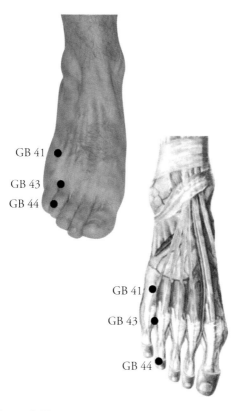

GB 41
GB 43
GB 44

GB 41
GB 43
GB 44

FIGURE 1.17

4 阳辅 (Yángfǔ) GB 38 Yang Support 经穴 Jing-river point of the gallbladder channel

Location: On the lateral aspect of the lower leg, 4 cun proximal to the tip of the lateral malleolus, slightly anterior to the anterior border of the fibula.

Acupuncture: Insert the needle perpendicularly to a depth of 1.0–1.5 cun and stimulate until there is a sore, numb sensation in the local area spreading to the foot.

Moxibustion: Apply 3–5 moxa cones or needle-warming moxibustion or, alternatively, hold a moxa stick above the point for 10–20 minutes.

Functions:

- Expels wind and clears heat
- Activates the channel and alleviates pain
- Benefits the sinews and bones

Indications: Migraine and pain of the external canthus.

5 阳陵泉 (Yánglíngquán) GB 34 Yang Mound Spring 合穴 He-sea point of the gallbladder channel

Location: In the sitting position with the knee bent at 90° or in the supine position, the point is located in the depression anterior and inferior to the head of the fibula.

Acupuncture:

1. Insert the needle perpendicularly in the direction of SP 9 (yīn líng quán) to a depth of 1.0–3.0 cun and stimulate until there is a sore, numb sensation in the local area radiating downwards.

2. Insert the needle obliquely to a depth of 0.5–0.8 cun and stimulate until there is a sore, numb sensation in the local area.

Moxibustion: Apply 3–5 moxa cones or needle-warming moxibustion or, alternatively, hold a moxa stick above the point for 5–10 minutes.

Functions:

- Relaxes sinews and benefits the joints
- Activates the channel and alleviates pain
- Spreads liver and gallbladder qi
- Clears liver and gallbladder dampness and heat

Indications: Headache, tinnitus, deafness and eye pain. Asthma and cough. Incontinence and enuresis. Pain in the chest, hypochondrium and knee, weakness and numbness of the lower extremities and hemiplegia.

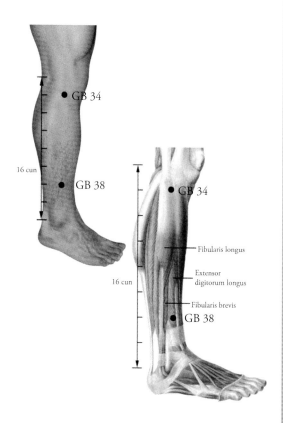

16 cun

GB 34

GB 38

Fibularis longus

Extensor
digitorum longus

Fibularis brevis

GB 38

FIGURE 1.18

Section X: Spleen Channel of Foot Taiyin; SP

1 隐白 (Yǐnbái) SP 1 Hidden White 井穴 Jing-well point of the spleen channel

Location: On the medial side of the big toe, 0.1 cun proximal and lateral to the corner of the nail.

Acupuncture:

1. Insert the needle to a depth of 0.1–0.2 cun until there is a sore, distending sensation in the local area.

2. Prick with a three-edged needle to bleed.

Moxibustion: Apply 3–7 moxa cones or hold a moxa stick above the point for 5–20 minutes.

Functions:

- Benefits qi and stops bleeding
- Invigorates the spleen
- Calms the spirit and restores consciousness

Indications: Irregular menstruation and metror-rhagia. Vomiting, blood in the stool and urine, hematochezia, abdominal distention, sudden and violent diarrhea and hernia. Epilepsy, insomnia with copious dreams, slow convulsions and fainting.

2 大都 (Dàdū) SP 2 Great Capital 荥穴 Ying-spring point of the spleen channel

Location: On the medial aspect of the foot, in a depression anterior and inferior to the proximal metatarsodigital joint of the big toe, at the junction where the skin changes texture.

Acupuncture: Insert the needle perpendicularly to a depth of 0.3–0.5 cun and sitmulate until there is a sore, numb sensation in the local area.

Moxibustion: Apply 1–3 moxa cones or hold a moxa stick above the point for 5–10 minutes. Prohibited during pregnancy up to 100 days after delivery.

Functions:

- Invigorates the spleen and harmonizes the middle heater
- Removes dampness and clears heat
- Alleviates pain
- Benefits spleen qi

Indications: Abdominal distention, pain and stomach ache.

3 太白 (Tàibái) SP 3 Great White 输穴 Shu-stream point of the spleen channel

Location: On the medial aspect of the foot, in the depression posterior and inferior to the proximal metatarsophalangeal joint of the big toe, at the junction where the skin changes texture.

Acupuncture: Insert the needle perpendicularly to a depth of 0.3–0.5 cun and stimulate until there is a sore, numb sensation in the local area.

Moxibustion: Apply 3–5 moxa cones or hold a moxa stick above the point for 5–10 minutes.

Functions:

- Invigorates the spleen
- Removes dampness and clears heat
- Harmonizes the spleen and stomach
- Clears heat and alleviates pain

Indications: Stomach ache, abdominal distention, pain and borborygmus. Metrorrhagia, irregular menstruation and insufficient lactation.

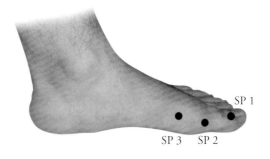

SP 1

SP 3   SP 2

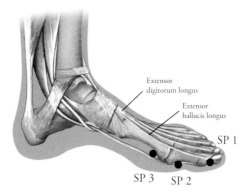

Extensor
digitorum longus

Extensor
hallucis longus

SP 1

SP 3   SP 2

FIGURE 1.19

4 商丘 (Shāngqiū) SP 5 Merchant Mound 经穴 Jing-river point of the spleen channel

Location: In the depression anterior and inferior to the medial malleolus, at the midpoint between the tuberosity of the navicular bone and the tip of the medial malleolus.

Acupuncture: Insert the needle perpendicularly to a depth of 0.3–0.5 cun and stimulate until there is a sore, numb sensation in the local area radiating to the ankle.

Moxibustion: Apply 3–5 moxa cones or hold a moxa stick above the point for 10–20 minutes.

Functions:

- Invigorates the spleen and resolves dampness
- Harmonizes the intestines and stomach
- Benefits the sinews and bones

Indications: Ankle pain.

5 阴陵泉 (Yīnlíngquán) SP 9
Yin Mound Spring 合穴 He-sea point of the spleen channel

Location: On the medial part of the lower leg, in the depression of the lower border of the medial condyle of the tibia.

Acupuncture: Insert the needle perpendicularly to a depth of 0.5–1.0 and stimulate until there is a sensation in the local area.

Moxibustion: Apply 3–5 moxa cones or needle-warming moxibustion or, alternatively, hold a moxa stick above the point for 5–10 minutes.

Functions:

- Removes dampness and clears heat
- Regulates the spleen and stomach
- Tonifies kidney and regulates menstruation
- Regulates the fluid passages
- Benefits the lower heater

Indications: Abdominal pain and distention. Edema, incontinence, enuresis, spermatorrhea and impotence. Irregular menstruation, dysmenorrhea and leucorrhea.

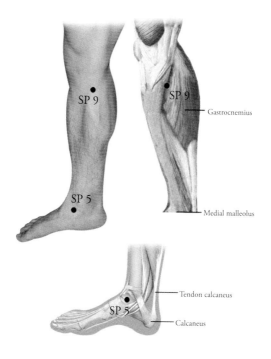

Gastrocnemius

Medial malleolus

Tendon calcaneus

Calcaneus

FIGURE 1.20

Section XI: Kidney Channel of Foot Shaoyin; KI

1 涌泉 (Yǒngquán) KI 1 Gushing Spring 井穴 Jing-well point of the kidney channel

Location: In a depression appearing on the sole, when the foot is in plantar flexion, approximately at the junction of the anterior and middle ⅓ of the sole (measured from the base of the 2nd toe to the back of the heel), between the 2nd and 3rd metatarsal.

Acupuncture: Insert the needle perpendicularly to a depth of 0.5–1.0 cun and stimulate until there is a sore, numb sensation in the local area spreading around the sole of the foot.

Moxibustion: Apply 3–7 moxa cones or hold a moxa stick above the point for 5–10 minutes.

Functions:
- Tonifies and nourishes the kidney
- Calms the liver to extinguish wind
- Calms the spirit and revives consciousness

Indications: Loss of consciousness, mania, epilepsy, infantile convulsions and headache. Sore throat and asthma. Enuresis.

2 然谷 (Rángǔ) KI 2 Burning Valley 荥穴 Ying-spring point of the kidney channel

Location: On the medial aspect of the foot, below the tuberosity of the navicular bone, at the junction where the skin changes texture.

Acupuncture: Insert the needle perpendicularly to a depth of 0.5–1.0 cun and stimulate until there is a sore, numb sensation in the local area spreading around the sole.

Moxibustion: Apply 3–5 moxa cones or hold a moxa stick above the point for 5–10 minutes.

Functions:

- Tonifies and nourishes the kidney
- Clears deficient heat
- Clears heat and regulates lower heater
- Benefits the bladder

Indications: Irregular menstruation, prolapse of the uterus, amenorrhea, dysmenorrhea, morbid leucorrhea, metrorrhagia and infertility.

3 太溪 (Tàixī) KI 3 Great Valley 输穴 Shu-stream point of the kidney channel

Location: On the medial aspect of the foot, posterior to the medial malleolus, in the depression between the tip of the medial malleolus and the tendon calcaneus.

Acupuncture: Insert the needle perpendicularly toward BL 60 (kūn lún) to a depth of 0.5–1.0 cun and stimulate until there is a sore, numb sensation in the local area.

Moxibustion: Apply 3–5 moxa cones or hold a moxa stick above the point for 5–10 minutes.

Functions:

- Nourishes kidney yin and clears deficient heat
- Tonifies kidney yang
- Tonifies the spleen and benefits the lung
- Strengthens the lumbar region

Indications: Enuresis, spermatorrhea, impotence and edema. Irregular menstruation, morbid leucorrhea and infertility. Cough, asthma and hemoptysis. Insomnia, amnesia and neurosis. Headache, tooth ache, sore throat, a sudden loss of voice, tinnitus and deafness. Soreness and swelling of the internal malleolus and pain of the heel.

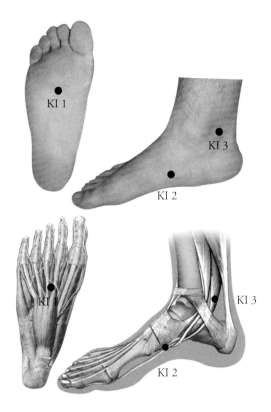

Figure 1.21

4 复溜 (Fùliū) KI 7 Returning Current 经穴 Jing-river point of the kidney channel

Location: On the medial aspect of the lower leg, 2 cun directly superior to KI 3 (tài xī), anterior to the tendon calcaneus.

Acupuncture: Insert the needle perpendicularly to a depth of 0.8–1.0 cun and stimulate until there is a sore, distending sensation in the local area.

Moxibustion: Apply 3–5 moxa cones or needle-warming moxibustion or, alternatively, hold a herbal moxa stick above the point for 10–15 minutes.

Functions:

- Tonifies the kidney and benefits the lumbar region
- Regulates the fluid passages and treats edema
- Regulates sweating and clears deficient heat

Indications: Night sweating and febrile disease without sweating.

5 阴谷 (Yīngǔ) KI 10 Yin Valley 合穴 He-sea point of the kidney channel

Location: On the medial aspect of the popliteal fossa when the knee is flexed, between the tendons of the muscles semitendinusus and semimembranosus.

Acupuncture: Insert the needle perpendicularly to a depth of 0.8–1.2 cun and stimulate until there is a sore, numb sensation in the local area.

Moxibustion: Apply 3–5 moxa cones or needle-warming moxibustion or, alternatively, hold a moxa stick above the point for 5–10 minutes.

Functions:

- Tonifies the kidney and benefits yang
- Benefits the lower heater
- Activates the channel and alleviates pain

Indications: Spermatorrhea and impotence. Irregular menstruation.

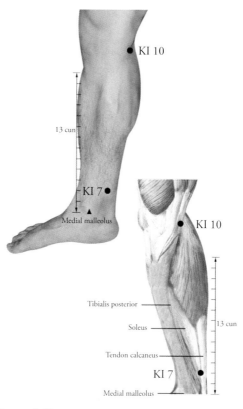

FIGURE 1.22

KI 10

13 cun

KI 7

Medial malleolus

KI 10

Tibialis posterior

Soleus

Tendon calcaneus

KI 7

Medial malleolus

13 cun

Section XII: Liver Channel of Foot Jueyin; LV

1 大敦 (Dàdūn) LV 1 Large Hill 井穴 Jing-well point of the liver channel

Location: On the foot, 0.1 cun proximal and lateral to the corner of the nail of the big toe.

Acupuncture:

1. Insert the needle subcutaneously to a depth of 0.1–0.2 cun and stimulate until there is a sore, numb sensation in the local area.

2. Prick with a three-edged needle to bleed.

Moxibustion: Apply 3–5 moxa cones or hold a moxa stick above the point for 5–10 minutes.

Functions:

- Regulates the uterus and bladder
- Regulates liver qi and stops menstrual bleeding

- Revives consciousness and calms the spirit
- Treats hernia

Indications: Amenorrhea, metrorrhagia, and prolapse of the uterus. Hernia, enuresis and disuria. Epilepsy.

2 行间 (Xíngjiān) LV 2 Active Interval 荥穴 Ying-spring point of the liver channel

Location: On the dorsum of the foot, proximal to the margin of the web between the 1st and 2nd toes, at the junction where the skin changes texture.

Acupuncture: Insert the needle subcutaneously to a depth of 0.1–0.2 cun and stimulate until there is a sore, numb sensation in the local area radiating to the dorsum of the foot.

Moxibustion: Apply 3–5 moxa cones or hold a moxa stick above the point for 5–10 minutes.

Functions:

- Clears liver fire and spreads liver qi
- Pacifies liver wind and relaxes the sinews
- Clears heat and calms the spirit
- Cools the blood and stops bleeding

Indications: Headache, pain and redness of the eyes, deviation of the mouth, tinnitus and deafness. Dizziness, stroke and epilepsy. Spermatorrhea and impotence. Dysmenorrhea, metrorrhagia, dysmenorrheal and morbid leucorrhea.

3 太冲 (Tàichōng) LV 3 Great Rushing 输穴 Shu-stream point of the liver channel

Location: On the dorsum of the foot, in the depression proximal to the 1st and 2nd metatarsophalangeal joints.

Acupuncture:

1. Insert the needle obliquely upwards to a depth of 0.5–1.0 cun and stimulate until there is a sore, numb sensation in the local area radiating to the sole of the foot.

2. Insert the needle obliquely outward to a depth of 1.0–1.5 cun and stimulate until there is a sore, numb sensation in the local area.

Moxibustion: Apply 3–5 moxa cones or needle-warming moxibustion or, alternatively, hold a moxa stick above the point for 10–20 minutes.

Functions:

- Clears liver fire and spreads liver qi
- Subdues liver yang and pacifies wind
- Nourishes liver blood and liver yin
- Clears the head and eyes
- Clears dampness and heat of liver and gallbladder
- Regulates menstruation

Indications: Headache and pain in the eye. Congestion in the chest. Vomiting. Enuresis. Irregular menstruation, dysmenorrhea, amenorrhea, metrorrhagia, metrostaxis, morbid leucorrhea and mastitis. Infantile convulsions, epilepsy, dizziness, irritability, insomnia and high blood pressure.

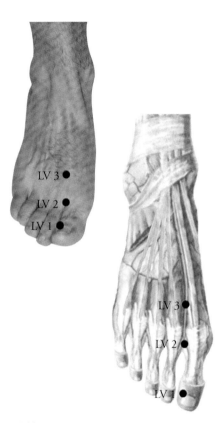

FIGURE 1.23

4 中封 (Zhōngfēng) LV 4
Mound Center 经穴 Jing-river point of the liver channel

Location: On the dorsum of the foot, anterior to the medial malleolus, between SP 5 (shāng qiū) and ST 41 (jiě xī), in the depression on the medial border of the tendon of the muscle tibilis anterior.

Acupuncture: Insert the needle perpendicularly to a depth of 0.5–0.8 cun and stimulate until there is a sore, numb sensation in the local area radiating to the toe.

Moxibustion: Apply 3–5 moxa cones or needle-warming moxibustion or, alternatively, hold a moxa stick above the point for 5–10 minutes.

Functions:

- Spreads the liver and regulates qi
- Clears liver and gallbladder heat
- Activates the channel and relaxes sinews

Indications: Hernia, pain of the external genitalia, spermatorrhea, lumbago and dysuria. Pain and swelling of the medial malleolus.

5 曲泉 (Qūquán) LV 8
Crooked Spring 合穴 He-sea
point of the liver channel

Location: On the medial aspect of the knee, in the depression on the medial end of the transverse popliteal crease when the knee is flexed, on the posterior border of the medial epicondyle of the femur, on the anterior portion of the insertion of the muscles semitendinosus and semimembranosus.

Acupuncture: Insert the needle perpendicularly to a depth of 1.0–1.5 cun and stimulate until there is a sore, numb sensation in the local area spreading to the knee joint and radiating to the foot.

Moxibustion: Apply 3–5 moxa cones or needle-warming moxibustion or, alternatively, hold a moxa stick above the point for 5–10 minutes.

Functions:

- Spreads liver qi
- Regulates menstruation and alleviates pain
- Clears dampness and heat and tonifies the bladder
- Invigorates blood and benefits the uterus

Indications: Irregular menstruation, dysmenorrhea, morbid leucorrhea. Hernia, impotence, spermatorrhea and dysuria.

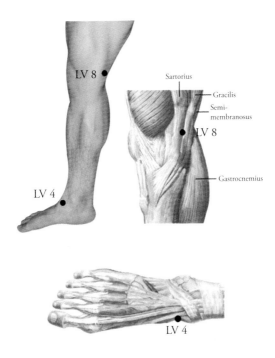

LV 8

Sartorius

Gracilis

Semi-membranosus

LV 8

Gastrocnemius

LV 4

LV 4

FIGURE 1.24

CHAPTER 2

Yuan-Source Points

1太渊 (Tàiyuān) LU 9 Supreme Abyss 肺经原穴 Yuan-source point of the lung channel

Location: On the transverse wrist crease, on the radial side of the radial artery where the radial pulse is palpable.

Acupuncture:

1. Insert the needle perpendicularly to a depth of 0.2–0.3 cun and stimulate until there is a numb, distending sensation in the local area.

2. Avoid puncturing the radial artery.

Moxibustion: Apply 1–3 moxa cones or hold a moxa stick above the point for 5–10 minutes. Scarring moxibustion is not applicable since the radial artery is located nearby.

Functions:

- Alleviates cough and transforms phlegm
- Descends lung qi
- Regulates and harmonizes the vessels
- Activates the channel and alleviates pain
- Tonifies qi and invigorates the spleen

Indications: Pain in the wrist and pulseless disease (Takayasu's arteritis).

2 神门 (Shénmén) HT 7 Spirit Door 心经原穴 Yuan-source point of the heart channel

Location: On the transverse crease of the wrist on the radial side of the tendon of the muscle flexor carpi ulnaris.

Acupuncture:

1. Insert the needle perpendicularly to a depth of 0.3–0.5 cun and stimulate until there is a sore, numbness in the local area with a sensation of electricity radiating to the fingers.

2. Insert the needle obliquely towards HT 4 (língdào) to a depth of 1.0–1.5 cun and stimulate until there is a sore, numb sensation in the local area radiating to the upper arm.

Moxibustion: Apply 1–3 moxa cones or hold a moxa stick above the point for 5–15 minutes.

Functions:

- Clears heat and calms the spirit
- Regulates and tonifies the heart

Indications: Irritability, amnesia, insomnia, loss of consciousness and epilepsy. Cardiac pain and palpitations.

3 大陵 (Dàlíng) PC 7 Great Mound
心包经原穴 Yuan-source point
of the pericardium channel

Location: On the palmar aspect of the forearm, in the middle of the transverse crease of the wrist.

Acupuncture:

1. Insert the needle perpendicularly to a depth of 0.3–0.5 cun and stimulate until

there is a sore, numbness in the local area with a sensation of electricity radiating to the finger tip.

2. Insert the needle perpendicularly into the wrist and stimulate until there is a sore, numb sensation in the local area.

3. Prick with a three-edged needle to bleed.

Moxibustion: Apply 3–5 moxa cones or hold a moxa stick above the point for 10–20 minutes.

Functions:

*   Descends rebellious qi and regulates the stomach
*   Clears heart heat and calms the spirit
*   Relieves congestion in the chest and regulates qi
*   Activates the channel and cools blood

Indications: Cardiac pain, palpitations and irritability.

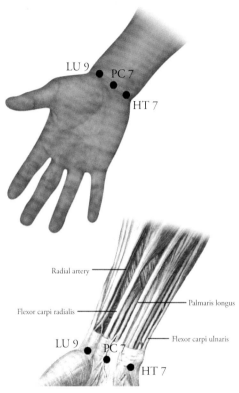

LU 9 PC 7

HT 7

Radial artery

Palmaris longus

Flexor carpi radialis

Flexor carpi ulnaris

LU 9 PC 7

HT 7

FIGURE 2.1

4 腕骨 (Wàngǔ) SI 4 Wrist Bone
小肠经原穴 Yuan-source point of the small intestine channel

Location: On the ulnar side of the palm, in the depression between the base of the 5th metacarpal bone and the hamate bone, at the junction where the skin changes texture.

Acupuncture: Insert the needle perpendicularly to a depth of 0.3–0.5 cun and stimulate until there is a sore, numb sensation in the local area spreading to the palm.

Moxibustion: Apply 3–5 moxa cones or needle-warming moxibustion or, alternatively, hold a moxa stick above the point for 5–10 minutes.

Functions:

- Activates the channel and alleviates pain
- Clears damp-heat and treats jaundice
- Clears heat and reduces swelling
- Regulates the small intestine

Indications: Headache and tinnitus. Pain in the fingers. Febrile conditions, jaundice, anhidrosis and malaria.

5 阳池 (Yángchí) TH 4 Pool of Yang 三焦经原穴 Yuan-source point of three heater channel

Location: On the dorsum aspect of the transverse wrist crease, in the depression on the ulnar side of the tendon of the muscle extensor digitorum communis.

Acupuncture:

1. Insert the needle perpendicularly to a depth of 0.3–0.5 cun and stimulate until there is a sore, distending sensation in the local area radiating to the middle finger.

2. Insert the needle subcutaneously to a depth of 0.5–1.0 cun and stimulate until there is a sore, numb sensation in the local area radiating to the wrist.

Moxibustion: Apply 3–5 moxa cones or needle-warming moxibustion or, alternatively, hold a moxa stick above the point for 3–5 minutes.

Functions:

- Clears wind and heat of the shaoyang channel
- Activates the channel and alleviates pain

Indications: Headache, dizziness, tinnitus, deafness, pain in the eyes, sore throat and thirst.

6 合谷 (Hégǔ) LI 4 Joining Valley 大肠经原穴 Yuan-source point of large intestine channel

Location: On the dorsum of the hand, between the 1st and 2nd metacarpal bones, on the radial side at the center of the 2nd metacarpal bone.

Acupuncture:

1. Insert the needle perpendicularly to a depth of 0.5–1.0 cun and stimulte until there is a sore, numb sensation in the local area radiating to the elbow, shoulder and face.

2. Insert the needle to a depth of 2.0 cun and stimulate until there is a sore, numb sensation in the palm radiating to the end of the fingers.

3. Insert the needle at LI 4 (hé gǔ) until it reaches the points PC 8 (láo gōng) or SI 3 (hòu xī) and stimulate until there is a sore, numb sensation radiating to the palm and the tip of the finger.

Moxibustion: Apply 5–9 moxa cones or needle-warming moxibustion or, alternatively, hold a moxa stick above the point for 10–20 minutes.

Functions:

- Relieves the surface and clears heat
- Regulates defensive qi and adjusts sweating
- Expels wind and releases the exterior
- Regulates the face, eyes, nose, mouth and ears
- Activates the channel and alleviates pain
- Induces labor

Indications: Headache, nasal obstruction, epistaxis, rhinorrhea, deafness, tinnitus, redness, swelling and pain in the eyes, tooth ache, mouth ulcers, jaw lock, deviation of the eye and mouth and soreness of the tongue. Stomach ache, abdominal pain, constipation and dysentery. Irregular menstruation, dysmenorrhea, amenorrhea, excessive excretion of the lochia, retention of the placenta and insufficient lactation. Spasms in the fingers, finger rigidity, pain of the arm and paralysis of the upper limbs. Fever, a cold sensation after sweating and hiccups.

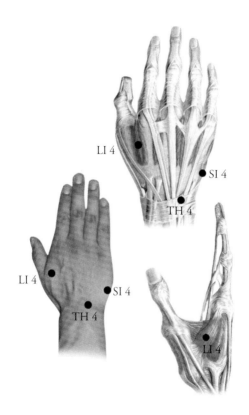

LI 4

SI 4

TH 4

LI 4

SI 4

TH 4

LI 4

FIGURE 2.2

7 太冲 (Tàichōng) LV 3 Great Rushing 肝经原穴 Yuan-source point of the liver channel

Location: On the dorsum of the foot, in the depression proximal to the 1st and 2nd metatarsophalangeal joints.

Acupuncture:

1. Insert the needle obliquely upwards to a depth of 0.5–1.0 cun and stimulate until there is a sore, numb sensation in the local area radiating to the sole of the foot.

2. Insert the needle obliquely outward to a depth of 1.0–1.5 cun and stimulate until there is a sore, numb sensation in the local area.

Moxibustion: Apply 3–5 moxa cones or needle-warming moxibustion or, alternatively, hold a moxa stick above the point for 10–20 minutes.

Functions:

- Clears liver fire and spreads liver qi
- Subdues liver yang and pacifies wind

- Nourishes liver blood and liver yin
- Clears the head and eyes
- Clears dampness and heat of liver and gallbladder
- Regulates menstruation

Indications: Headache and pain in the eyes. Congestion of the chest. Vomiting. Enuresis. Irregular menstruation, dysmenorrhea, amenorrhea, metrorrhagia, metrostaxis, morbid leucorrhea and mastitis. Infantile convulsions, epilepsy, dizziness, irritability, insomnia and high blood pressure.

8 冲阳 (Chōngyáng) ST 42 Rushing Yang 胃经原穴 Yuan-source point of the stomach channel

Location: On the dorsum of the foot, between the tendon of the muscles extensor pollicis longus and extensor digitorum longus where the pulse of the dorsal artery can be felt.

Acupuncture:

1. Insert the needle perpendicularly to a depth of 0.2–0.3 cun.

2. Avoid puncturing the artery.

Moxibustion: Apply 3–5 moxa cones or hold a moxa stick above the point for 5–10 minutes.

Functions:

- Harmonizes the stomach and transforms phlegm
- Activates the channel and alleviates pain
- Calms the spirit

Indications: Vomiting, stomach ache and a poor appetite. Manic psychosis and epilepsy. Paralysis of the foot.

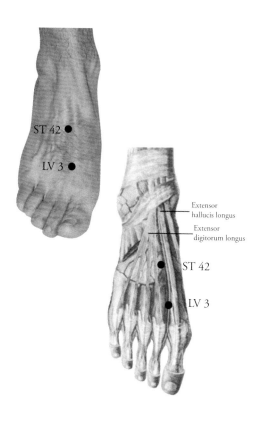

ST 42

LV 3

Extensor
hallucis longus

Extensor
digitorum longus

ST 42

LV 3

FIGURE 2.3

9 京骨 (Jīnggǔ) BL 64 Capital Bone 膀胱经原穴 Yuan-source point of the bladder channel

Location: On the lateral side of the foot, inferior to the tuberosity of the 5th metatarsal bone, at the junction where the skin changes texture.

Acupuncture: Insert the needle perpendicularly to a depth of 0.3–0.5 cun and stimulate until there is a sore, numb sensation in the local area.

Moxibustion: Apply 3–7 moxa cones or needle-warming moxibustion or, alternatively, hold a moxa stick above the point for 5–10 minutes.

Functions:

- Relaxes sinews, activates the channel and alleviates pain
- Clears heat and expels wind
- Calms the spirit

Indications: Headache and lumbago.

10 丘墟 (Qiūxū) GB 40 Eminent Region 胆经原穴 Yuan-source point of the gallbladder

Location: Anterior and inferior to the external malleolus, in the depression on the lateral aspect of the tendon of the muscle extensor digitorum longus.

Acupuncture:

1. Insert the needle perpendicularly to a depth of 1.0–1.5 cun and stimulate until there is a sore, numb sensation in the local area spreading to the foot.

2. Insert the needle obliquely outward to BL 62 (shēn mài) to a depth of 0.8–1.2 cun and stimulate until there is a sore and numb sensation in the local area spreading to the ankle.

Moxibustion: Apply 5–7 moxa cones or needle-warming moxibustion or, alternatively, hold a moxa stick above the point for 10–20 minutes.

Functions:

- Clears dampness and treats jaundice
- Clears heat and relaxes the sinews
- Clears gallbladder dampness and heat
- Activates the channel and benefits the joints

Indications: Migraine, eye conditions, tooth ache, deafness, sore throat and neck pain. Amenorrhea. Malaria and hernia.

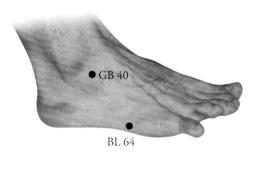

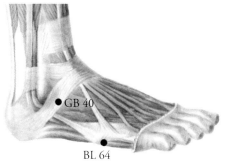

FIGURE 2.4

11 太白 (Tàibái) SP 3 Great White 脾经原穴 Yuan-source point of the spleen channel

Location: On the medial side of foot, in the depression posterior and inferior to the proximal metatarsophalangeal joint of the big toe, at the junction where the skin changes texture

Acupuncture: Insert the needle perpendicularly to a depth of 0.3–0.5 cun and stimulate until there is a sore, numb sensation in the local area.

Moxibustion: Apply 3–5 moxa cones or hold a moxa stick above the point for 5–10 minutes.

Functions:

- Invigorates the spleen
- Removes dampness and clears heat
- Harmonizes the spleen and stomach
- Clears heat and alleviates pain

Indications: Stomach ache, borborygmus, abdominal distention and pain. Metrorrhagia, irregular menstruation and insufficient lactation.

12 太溪 (Tàixī) KI 3 Great Valley 肾经原穴 Yuan-source point of the kidney channel

Location: On the medial aspect of the foot, posterior to the medial malleolus, in the depression between the tip of the medial malleolus and the tendon calcaneus.

Acupuncture: Insert the needle perpendicularly toward BL 60 (kūnlún) to a depth of 0.5–1.0 cun and stimulate until there is a sore, numb sensation in the local area.

Moxibustion: Apply 3–5 moxa cones or hold a moxa stick above the point for 5–10 minutes.

Functions:

- Nourishes kidney yin and clears deficient heat
- Tonifies kidney yang
- Tonifies spleen and benefits lung
- Strengthens the lumbar region

Indications: Enuresis, spermatorrhea, impotence and edema. Irregular menstruation, morbid leucorrhea and infertility. Cough, asthma and hemoptysis. Insomnia, amnesia and neurosis. Headache, tooth ache, sore throat, sudden loss of voice, tinnitus and deafness. Soreness and swelling of the internal malleolus and pain in the heel.

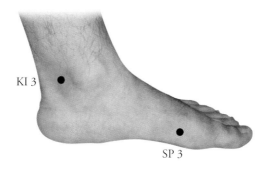

KI 3

SP 3

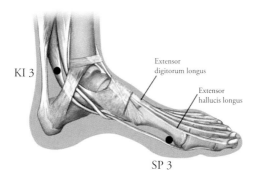

KI 3

Extensor
digitorum longus

Extensor
hallucis longus

SP 3

FIGURE 2.5

CHAPTER 3
Luo-Connecting Points

1 列缺 (Lièquē) LU 7 Broken Sequence 肺经络穴 Luo-connecting point of the lung channel

Location: On the radial side of the forearm, 1.5 cun proximal to the transverse crease of the wrist, superior to the styloid process of the radius and between tendons of the muscles brachioradialis and abductor pollicis longus.

Acupuncture:

1. Insert the needle obliquely upwards to a depth of 0.2–0.3 cun and stimulate until there is a sore, heavy and numb sensation in the local area radiating to the elbow and the shoulder.

2. Insert the needle obliquely downwards to a depth of 0.3–0.5 cun and stimulate until there is a sensation in the local area.

Moxibustion: Apply 3–5 moxa cones or hold a moxa stick above the point for 5–10 minutes. Scarring moxibustion is not applicable since the skin is very thin at this point.

Functions:

- Releases the exterior and expels wind
- Regulates the conception vessel
- Regulates the fluid passageways
- Activates the channel and alleviates pain
- Promotes the descending functions of the lung
- Benefits the head and nape

Indications: Cough, sore throat, asthma and shortness of breath. Headache, migraine and neck stiffness.

2 通里 (Tōnglǐ) HT 5 Internal Communication 心经络穴 Luo-connecting point of the heart channel

Location: On the palmar aspect of the forearm, on a line connecting HT 7 (shénmén) to HT 3 (shàohǎi), 1 cun proximal to HT 7 (shénmén).

Acupuncture: Insert the needle perpendicularly to a depth of 0.3–0.5 cun and stimulate until there is a sore, numb sensation in the local area radiating down the heart channel and reaching the ring or little finger, or reaching the head and chest.

Moxibustion: Apply 1–3 moxa cones or hold a moxa stick above the point for 10–20 minutes.

Functions:

- Calms the spirit
- Activates the channel and alleviates pain
- Benefits the throat and tongue

Indications: Cardiac pain and shock.

3 内关 (Nèiguān) PC 6 Inner Gate 心包经络穴 Luo-connecting point of the pericardium channel

Location: On the palmar aspect of the forearm, 2 cun proximal to the transverse crease of the wrist, on the line connecting PC 3 (qūzé) to PC 7 (dàlíng).

Acupuncture: Insert the needle perpendicularly to a depth of 0.3–0.5 cun and stimulate until there is a sore and numb sensation in the local area radiating down the heart channel and reaching the ring or little finger, or reaching the head and chest.

Moxibustion: Apply 1–3 moxa cones or hold a moxa stick above the point for 10–20 minutes.

Functions:

- Calms the spirit
- Activates the channel and alleviates pain
- Benefits the throat and tongue

Indications: Cardiac pain, palpitations and insomnia. Chest distention and asthma. Stomach ache, vomiting and hiccupping.

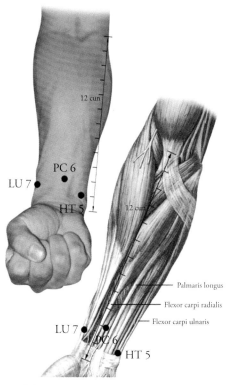

12 cun

PC 6

LU 7

HT 5

12 cun

Palmaris longus

Flexor carpi radialis

Flexor carpi ulnaris

LU 7

PC 6

HT 5

FIGURE 3.1

4 偏历 (Piānlì) LI 6 Side Passage
大肠经络穴 Luo-connecting
point of large intestine channel

Location: On the radial side of the posterior forearm, 3 cun proximal to the wrist crease, on the line connecting LI 5 (yángxī) and LI 11 (qǔchí) when the elbow is flexed.

Acupuncture:

1. Insert the needle perpendicularly to a depth of 0.3–0.5 cun and stimulate until there is a sore, numb sensation in the local area.

2. Insert the needle obliquely towards the elbow to a depth of 0.5–0.8 cun and stimulate until there is a sore, numb sensation in the local area radiating to the forearm and the elbow.

Moxibustion: Apply 3–5 moxa cones or needle-warming moxibustion or, alternatively, hold a moxa stick above the point for 5–10 minutes.

Functions:

- Clears heat and promotes diuresis
- Regulates the fluid passageways

- Dredges the channel

Indications: Deafness, tinnitus, sore throat, nosebleed, swelling of the cheeks. Dysuria.

5 支正 (Zhīzhèng) SI 7 Branch of the Upright 小肠经络穴 Luo-connecting point of the small intestine channel

Location: On the anterior border of the ulnar, on the line connecting SI 5 (yánggǔ) to SI 8 (xiǎohǎi), 5 cun proximal to the posterior transverse wrist crease.

Acupuncture: Insert the needle perpendicularly or obliquely to a depth of 0.5–1.0 cun and stimulate until there is a distending and heavy sensation radiating to the hand.

Moxibustion: Apply 3–5 moxa cones or needle-warming moxibustion or, alternatively, hold a moxa stick above the point for 5–10 minutes.

Functions:

- Clears heat and calms the spirit
- Activates the channel and alleviates pain

Indications: Headache, dizziness, manic psychosis and epilepsy. Pain in the elbow and fingers, and neck stiffness. Febrile disease.

6 外关 (Wàiguān) TH 5 Outer Gate 三焦经络穴 Luo-connecting point of the three heater channel

Location: On the dorsal aspect of the forearm, on the line connecting TH 4 (yangchí) to the tip of the elbow, 2 cun proximal to the transverse crease of the wrist, in the depression between the ulna and radius.

Acupuncture:

1. Insert the needle perpendicularly to a depth of 0.5–1.0 cun and stimulate until there is a sore, numb sensation in the local area radiating to the tip of the finger.

2. Insert the needle obliquely to a depth of 1.5–2.0 cun and stimulate until there is a sore, numb sensation in the local area radiating to the elbow and shoulder.

Moxibustion: Apply 3–5 moxa cones or needle-warming moxibustion or, alternatively, hold a moxa stick above the point for 3–5 minutes.

Functions:

- Expels wind, clears heat and releases the exterior
- Opens the yang linking vessel
- Activates the channel and alleviates pain

Indications: Headache, tinnitus, tooth ache and redness, swelling and pain of the eyes. Pain in the upper extremities. Febrile diseases.

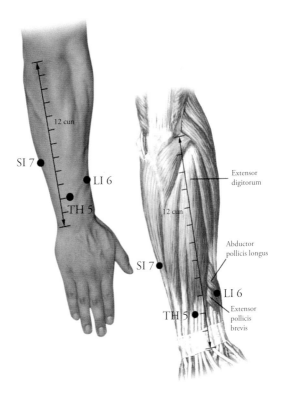

FIGURE 3.2

7 丰隆 (Fēnglóng) ST 40 Prosperous Abundance 胃经络穴 Luo-connecting point of the stomach channel

Location: 8 cun superior to the tip of the lateral malleolus, two finger's width lateral from the anterior ridge of the tibia.

Acupuncture:

1. Insert the needle perpendicularly to a depth of 1.0–1.5 cun and stimulate until there is a sensation radiating to the foot and the 2nd and 3rd toes.

2. Insert the needle obliquely upwards and stimulate until there is a sensation radiating to ST 31 (bìguān), ST 25 (tiānshū), and even ST 12 (quēpén) and ST 8 (tóuwéi).

Moxibustion: Apply 5–7 moxa cones or needle-warming moxibustion or, alternatively, hold a moxa stick above the point for 10–20 minutes.

Functions:

- Transforms phlegm and dampness
- Harmonizes the intestines and stomach
- Nourishes the spleen

- Clears phlegm in the lung and alleviates cough and wheezing
- Clears phlegm of the heart and calms the spirit
- Activates the channel and alleviates pain

Indications: Hiccupping, vomiting, stomach ache, constipation and difficult urination. Epilepsy, headache and dizziness. Asthma and sore throat.

8 飞扬 (Fēiyáng) BL 58 Flying Yang 膀胱经络穴 Luo-connecting point of the bladder channel

Location: On the posterior aspect of the lower leg, posterior to the external malleolus, 7 cun superior to BL 60 (kūnlún), 1 cun inferior and lateral to BL 57 (chéngshān).

Acupuncture: Insert the needle perpendicularly to a depth of 0.7–1.0 cun and stimulate until there is a sore, numb sensation in the local area.

Moxibustion: Apply 3–5 moxa cones or needle-warming moxibustion or, alternatively, hold a moxa stick above the point for 5–10 minutes.

Functions:

- Relaxes the sinews, activates the channel and alleviates pain
- Expels wind of the taiyang channel and clears heat

Indications: Headache, dizziness and epistaxis. Neck stiffness, pain in the legs and waist and weakness of the knees.

9 光明 (Guāngmíng) GB 37 Bright Light 胆经络穴 Luo-connecting point of the gallbladder channel

Location: On the lateral aspect of the lower leg, 5 cun proximal to the tip of the external malleolus, on the anterior border of the fibula, between the muscles extensor digitorum longus and peroneus brevis.

Acupuncture: Insert the needle perpendicularly to a depth of 1.0–1.2 cun and stimulate until there is a sore, numb sensation in the local area radiating to the knee or the inside of the foot.

Moxibustion: Apply 3–5 moxa cones or needle-warming moxibustion or, alternatively, hold a moxa stick above the point for 10–20 minutes.

Functions:

- Spreads liver qi and benefits the eyes
- Activates the channel and alleviates pain
- Dispels wind and damp

Indications: Redness, swelling and pain of the eyes and blurred vision. Mastitis, muscular atrophy and numbness, flaccidity and pain in the lower limbs.

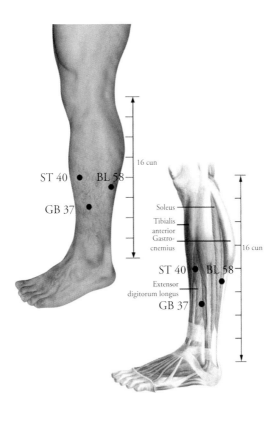

ST 40   BL 58

GB 37

16 cun

Soleus
Tibialis
anterior
Gastro-
cnemius

16 cun

ST 40   BL 58

Extensor
digitorum longus

GB 37

Figure 3.3

10 蠡沟 (Lígōu) LV 5 Calf Gutter 肝经络穴 Luo-connecting point of the liver channel

Location: On the medial aspect of the lower limb, 5 cun proximal to the tip of the medial malleolus, on the posterior border of the tibia.

Acupuncture: Insert the needle perpendicularly to a depth of 1.0–1.2 cun and stimulate until there is a sore, numb sensation in the local area radiating to the knee or the inside of the foot.

Moxibustion: Apply 3–5 moxa cones or needle-warming moxibustion or, alternatively, hold a moxa stick above the point for 10–20 minutes.

Functions:

- Spreads liver qi and benefits the eyes
- Activates the channel and alleviates pain
- Dispels wind and damp

Indications: Enuresis. Irregular menstruation, bloody and morbid leucorrhea, prolapse of the uterus, metrorrhagia and metrostaxis. Soreness and numbness of the foot and tibia.

11 公孙 (Gōngsūn) SP 4 Yellow Emperor 脾经络穴 Luo-connecting point of the spleen channel

Location: On the medial side of the foot, in the depression anterior and inferior to the base of the 1st metatarsal bone, at the junction where the skin changes texture.

Acupuncture: Insert the needle perpendicularly towards KI 1 (yǒngquán) to a depth of 0.5–0.8 cun and stimulate until there is a sore, numb sensation in the local area radiating to the sole of the foot.

Moxibustion: Apply 3–5 moxa cones or needle-warming moxibustion or, alternatively, hold a moxa stick above the point for 10–20 minutes.

Functions:

- Invigorates the spleen and harmonizes the middle heater
- Regulates qi and resolves dampness
- Regulates the penetrating and conception vessels
- Regulates qi

Indications: Vomiting, hiccups, abdominal pain and stomach ache.

12 大钟 (Dàzhōng) KI 4 Large Goblet 肾经络穴 Luo-connecting point of the kidney channel

Location: On the medial side of the foot, posterior and inferior to the medial malleolus, in the depression anterior to the border of the tendon calcaneus.

Acupuncture: Insert the needle perpendicularly to a depth of 0.5–1.0 cun and stimulate until there is a sore, numb sensation in the local area.

Moxibustion: Apply 3–5 moxa cones or needle-warming moxibustion or, alternatively, hold a moxa stick above the point for 5–10 minutes.

Functions:

- Tonifies the kidney
- Clears heat and calms the spirit
- Regulates menstruation

Indications: Disorders of the head and five sense organs. Sore throat.

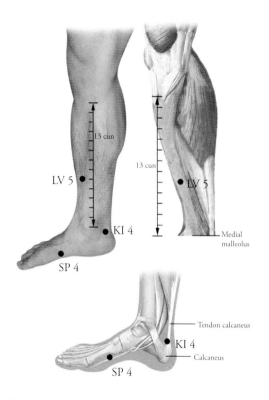

FIGURE 3.4

13 鸠尾 (Jiūwěi) CV 15 Dove's Tail 任脉络穴 Luo-connecting point of the conception vessel

Location: On the upper abdomen, on the anterior midline, 1 cun inferior to the sternocostal angle.

Acupuncture:

1. Insert the needle perpendicularly to a depth of 0.5–1.0 cun and stimulate until there is a sore, distending sensation in the local area.

2. Avoid deep needling to prevent injury to the heart and liver.

Moxibustion: Apply 3–5 moxa cones or hold a moxa stick above the point for 10–20 minutes.

Functions:

• Unbinds the chest and harmonizes the diaphragm

• Transforms phlegm and calms the spirit

- Harmonizes the stomach and descends rebellion

Indications: General pain of the chest and cardiac pain.

14 大包 (Dàbāo) SP 21 Great Wrapping 脾之大络 Great luo-connecting point of the spleen channel

Location: On the lateral aspect of the chest, on the mid-axillary line, 6 cun inferior to the center of the axilla, in the 6th intercostal space.

Acupuncture:

1. Insert the needle obliquely backwards to a depth of 0.5–0.8 cun and stimulate until there is a sore, numb sensation in the local area.

2. Insert the needle obliquely upwards and stimulate until there is a sore, numb sensation in the local area to treat neck sprains.

3. Avoid deep needling to prevent pneumo-thorax.

Moxibustion: Apply 3–5 moxa cones or hold a moxa stick above the point for 10–20 minutes.

Functions:

- Regulates qi and blood
- Relieves congestion in the chest and invigorates the spleen

Indications: Costal pain and asthma. Body aches and weakness of the limbs.

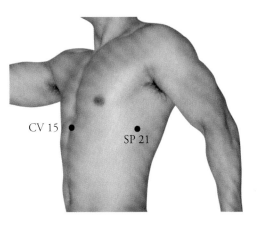

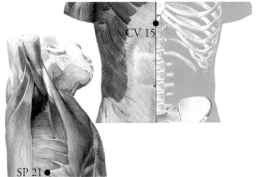

CV 15

SP 21

CV 15

SP 21

FIGURE 3.5

15 长强 (Chángqiáng) GV 1 Long Strength 督脉络穴 Luo-connecting point of the governing vessel

Location: Below the tip of the coccyx, at the midpoint between the tip of the coccyx and the anus.

Acupuncture:

1. Insert the needle obliquely to a depth of 0.5–1.0 cun proximally to the anterior border of the coccyx and stimulate until there is a sore, numb sensation in the local area radiating to the coccyx and the anus. Sometimes the sensation can spread to GV 4 (mìngmén) and GV 20 (bǎihuì).

2. Prick with a three-edged needle to bleed.

3. Avoid deep insertion to prevent puncturing the rectum.

Moxibustion: Moxibustion is prohibited.

Functions:

- Nourishes yin and descends yang
- Tonifies qi and calms the spirit
- Activates the channel and alleviates pain
- Treats hemorrhoids

Indications: Diarrhea, constipation, blood in the stools, hemorrhoids and prolapsus of the rectum. Spermatorrhea, impotence and pruritus perineum. Infantile epilepsy and manic psychosis. Pain in the coccyx and sacrum.

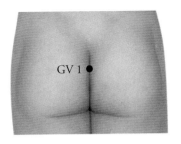

GV 1

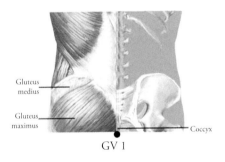

Gluteus medius

Gluteus maximus

Coccyx

GV 1

FIGURE 3.6

CHAPTER 4

Xi-Cleft Points

1 孔最 (Kǒngzuì) LU 6 Collection Hole 肺经郄穴 Xi-cleft point of the lung channel

Location: On the line connecting LU 9 (tàiyuān) and LU 5 (chǐzé), 7 cun above the transverse crease of the wrist on the palmar aspect of the forearm.

Acupuncture: Insert the needle perpendicularly to a depth of 0.5–0.8 cun and stimulate until there is a sore, numb and heavy sensation in the local area radiating to the forearm.

Moxibustion: Apply 5–7 moxa cones or needle-warming moxibustion or, alternatively, hold a moxa stick above the point for 10–20 minutes.

Functions:

- Clears heat and removes toxins
- Disperses and descends lung qi

- Clears heat and moisturizes the lung
- Clears heat and stops bleeding
- Relieves sore throat

Indications: Hemoptysis, epistaxis and sore thoat.

2 阴郄 (Yīnxì) HT 6 Yin Accummulation 心经郄穴 Xi-cleft point of the heart channel

Location: On the palmar aspect of the forearm, on a line connecting HT 7 (shénmén) to HT 3 (shàohǎi), 0.5 cun proximal to HT 7 (shénmén).

Acupuncture: Insert the needle perpendicularly to a depth of 0.5–0.8 cun and stimulate until there is a sore, numb and heavy sensation in the local area radiating to the forearm.

Moxibustion: Apply 5–7 moxa cones or needle-warming moxibustion or, alternatively, hold a moxa stick above the point for 10–20 minutes.

Functions:

- Clears heat and removes toxins
- Disperses and descends lung qi
- Clears heat and moisturizes the lung
- Clears heat and stops bleeding
- Relieves sore throat

Indications: Cardiac pain and shock. Coughing or vomiting blood. Irritability and night sweat.

3 郄门 (Xìmén) PC 4 Gate of Opposition 心包经郄穴 Xi-cleft point of the pericardium channel

Location: On the palmar side of the forearm, 5 cun superior to the transverse crease of the wrist, on the line connecting PC 3 (qūzé) to PC 7 (dàlíng).

Acupuncture: Insert the needle perpendicularly to a depth of 0.5–0.8 cun and stimulate until there is a sore, numb sensation in the local area radiating to the finger.

Moxibustion: Apply 3–5 moxa cones or hold a moxa stick above the point for 10–20 minutes.

Functions:

- Regulates qi and alleviates pain
- Activates blood circulation and dispels stasis
- Cools the blood and stops bleeding
- Calms the spirit

Indications: Cardiac pain and palpitation. Hemoptysis.

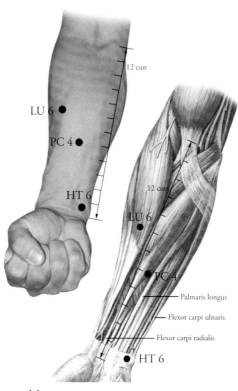

LU 6

PC 4

HT 6

12 cun

12 cun

LU 6

PC 4

Palmaris longus

Flexor carpi ulnaris

Flexor carpi radialis

HT 6

Figure 4.1

4 温溜 (Wēnliū) LI 7 Warm Current 大肠经郄穴 Xi-cleft point of the large intestine channel

Location: On the radial side of the arm, with the elbow flexed, the point is 5 cun proximal to the transverse crease of the wrist on the line connecting LI 5 (yángxī) and LI 11 (qǔchí).

Acupuncture: Insert the needle perpendicularly to a depth of 0.5–1.0 cun and stimulate until there is a sore, numb sensation in the local area radiating to the hand.

Moxibustion: Apply 3–5 moxa cones or needle-warming moxibustion or, alternatively, hold a moxa stick above the point for 5–10 minutes.

Functions:

- Clears heat and removes toxins
- Regulates and harmonizes the intestines and stomach
- Clears yangming fire

Indications: Headache, tooth ache and swelling of the pharynx. Pain of the shoulder and back, and paralysis of the upper limbs. Fever.

5 养老 (Yǎnglǎo) SI 6 Nourishing the Old 小肠经郄穴 Xi-cleft point of the small intestine channel

Location: On the ulnar aspect of the forearm, in the depression on the radial side of the styloid process of the ulna.

Acupuncture: Insert the needle obliquely upwards to a depth of 0.5–0.8 cun and stimulate until there is a sore, numb sensation in the wrist radiating to the shoulder and elbow.

Moxibustion: Apply 3–5 moxa cones or hold a moxa stick above the point for 10–20 minutes.

Functions:

- Activates the channel and alleviates pain
- Improves the vision
- Benefits the shoulders and arms

Indications: Hemiplegia and acute lumbago.

6 会宗 (Huìzōng) TH 7 三焦经郄穴 Xi-cleft point of the three heater channel

Location: On the dorsal aspect of the forearm, 3 cun proximal to the transverse wrist crease, in the depression between the ulna and radius, on the ulnar side of TH 6 (zhīgōu) and radial side of the ulna.

Acupuncture: Insert the needle perpendicularly to a depth of 0.5–1.0 cun and stimulate until there is a sore, numb sensation in the local area.

Moxibustion: Apply 3–5 moxa cones or needle-warming moxibustion or, alternatively, hold a moxa stick above the point for 5–10 minutes.

Functions:

- Activates the channel and alleviates pain
- Clears the shaoyang channel
- Clears heat and calms the spirit

Indications: Migraine, deafness and tinnitus.

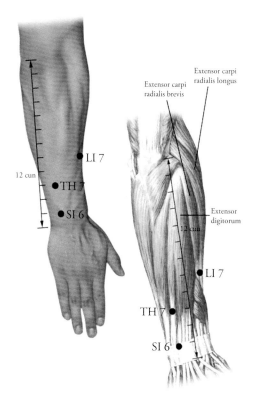

Extensor carpi radialis brevis

Extensor carpi radialis longus

Extensor digitorum

12 cun

LI 7

TH 7

SI 6

FIGURE 4.2

7 梁丘 (Liángqiū) ST 34 Beam Mound 胃经郄穴 Xi-cleft point of the stomach channel

Location: On the anterior aspect of the thigh, on the line connecting the anterior superior iliac spine and lateral border of the patella, 2 cun proximal to the patella when the knee is flexed.

Acupuncture: Insert the needle perpendicularly to a depth of 1.0–1.5 cun until there is a sore, numb sensation in the local area radiating to the knee.

Moxibustion: Apply 7–9 moxa cones or needle-warming moxibustion or, alternatively, hold a moxa stick above the point for 10–20 minutes.

Functions:

- Activates the channel and alleviates pain
- Harmonizes the stomach and regulates qi

Indications: Stomach ache, borborygmus and diarrhea. Knee pain.

8 水泉 (Shuǐquán) KI 5 Water Spring 肾经郄穴 Xi-cleft point of the kidney channel

Location: On the medial side of the foot, posterior and inferior to the medial malleolus, 1 cun directly inferior to KI 3 (tàixī), in the depression anterior to the tuberosity of the calcaneum.

Acupuncture: Insert the needle perpendicularly to a depth of 0.3–0.5 cun and stimulate until there is a sore, numb sensation in the local area radiating to the chest and abdomen.

Moxibustion: Apply 3–5 moxa cones or hold a moxa stick above the point for 5–10 minutes.

Functions:

- Regulates the penetrating and conception vessels
- Regulates menstruation

Indications: Irregular menstruation, amenorrhea and dysmenorrhea. Dysuria.

9 金门 (Jīnmén) BL 63 Golden Gate 膀胱经郄穴 Xi-cleft point of the bladder channel

Location: On the lateral side of the foot, inferior to the anterior border of the external malleolus, lateral to the lower border of the cuboid bone.

Acupuncture: Insert the needle perpendicularly to a depth of 0.3–0.5 cun and stimulate until there is a sore, numb sensation in the local area.

Moxibustion: Apply 3–5 moxa cones or needle-warming moxibustion or, alternatively, hold a moxa stick above the point for 5–10 minutes.

Functions:

- Relaxes the sinews, activates the channel and alleviates pain
- Calms the spirit

Indications: Headache and tooth ache.

10 外丘 (Wàiqiū) GB 36 External Region 胆经郄穴 Xi-cleft point of the gallbladder channel

Location: On the lateral aspect of the lower limb, 7 cun proximal to the tip of the external malleolus, on a level with GB 35 (yang jiāo), on the anterior border of the fibula.

Acupuncture: Insert the needle perpendicularly to a depth of 0.5–0.8 cun and stimulate until there is a sore, numb sensation in the local area radiating to the foot.

Moxibustion: Apply 3–5 moxa cones or needle-warming moxibustion or, alternatively, hold a moxa stick above the point for 5–10 minutes.

Functions:

- Clears and benefits liver and gallbladder qi
- Activates the channel and alleviates pain
- Clears heat and removes toxins

Indications: Congestion in the chest and the hypochondrium.

11 地机 (Dìjī) SP 8 Earth Pivot 脾经郄穴 Xi-cleft point of the spleen channel

Location: On the medial aspect of the lower leg, on the line connecting the medial malleolus to SP 9 (yīnlíngquán), 3 cun inferior to SP 9 (yīnlíngquán).

Acupuncture: Insert the needle perpendicularly to a depth of 1.0–1.5 cun and stimulate until there is a sore, numb sensation in the local area radiating to the calf.

Moxibustion: Apply 3–5 moxa cones or needle-warming moxibustion or, alternatively, hold a moxa stick above the point for 5–10 minutes.

Functions:

- Regulates menstruation and invigorates blood
- Harmonizes the spleen and resolves dampness
- Alleviates pain

Indications: A poor appetite and abdominal distention and pain. Edema, spermatorrhea and dysuria. Irregular menstruation and dysmenorrhea. Pain and numbness of the feet and legs.

12 中都 (Zhōngdū) LV 6
Central City 肝经郄穴 Xi-cleft point of the liver channel

Location: On the medial aspect of the lower leg, 7 cun proximal to the tip of the medial malleolus, on the medial border of the tibia.

Acupuncture: Insert the needle perpendicularly to a depth of 1.0–1.5 cun and stimulate until there is a sore, numb sensation in the local area radiating to the foot.

Moxibustion: Apply 3–5 moxa cones or needle-warming moxibustion or, alternatively, hold a moxa stick above the point for 5–10 minutes.

Functions:

- Regulates gallbladder qi and calms the spirit
- Activates the channel and alleviates pain

Indications: Abdominal distention. Hernia and spermatorrhea. Metrorrhagia and retention of lochia.

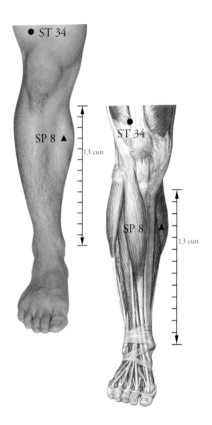

FIGURE 4.3

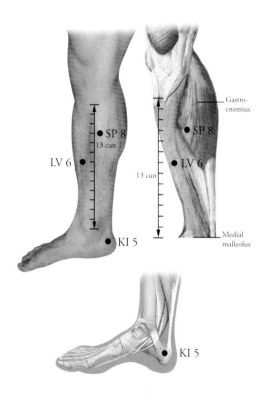

FIGURE 4.4

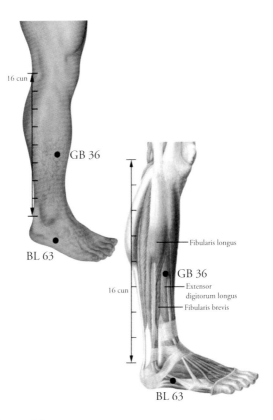

FIGURE 4.5

13 筑宾 (Zhùbīn) KI 9 House Guest 阴维郄穴 Xi-cleft point of the yin linking vessel

Location: On the medial aspect of the lower leg, on the line connecting KI 10 (yīngǔ) and KI 3 (tàixī), 5 cun superior to KI 3 (tàixī), medial and inferior to the belly of the muscle gastrocnemius.

Acupuncture: Insert the needle perpendicularly to a depth of 0.5–0.8 cun and stimulate until there is a sore, numb sensation in the local area radiating to either the thigh or the sole of the foot.

Moxibustion: Apply 3–5 moxa cones or needle-warming moxibustion or, alternatively, hold a moxa stick above the point for 5–10 minutes.

Functions:

- Tonifies and regulates liver and kidney
- Clears the heart and transforms phlegm.

Indications: Mania and epilepsy. Hernia. Pain on the medial aspect of the lower limbs.

14 交信 (Jiāoxìn) KI 8
Communicating Belief 阴跷郄穴 Xi-cleft point of the yin motility vessel

Location: On the medial aspect of the lower leg, 2 cun superior to KI 3 (tàixī), 0.5 cun anterior to KI 7 (fùliū), posterior to the medial border of the tibia.

Acupuncture: Insert the needle perpendicularly to a depth of 0.8–1.0 cun and stimulate until there is a sore, distending sensation in the local area.

Moxibustion: Apply 3–5 moxa cones or needle-warming moxibustion or, alternatively, hold a herbal moxa stick above the point for 10–15 minutes.

Functions:

- Regulates the conception and penetrating vessels
- Tonifies kidney and regulates menstruation
- Benefits the menstruation
- Clears dampness and heat

Indications: Irregular menstruation.

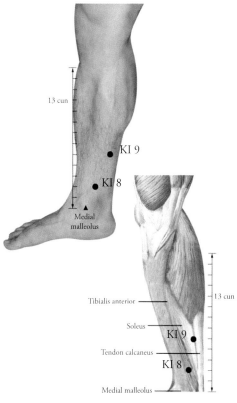

13 cun

KI 9

KI 8

Medial
malleolus

Tibialis anterior

Soleus

KI 9

Tendon calcaneus

KI 8

Medial malleolus

13 cun

FIGURE 4.6

15 阳交 (Yángjiāo) GB 35 Yang Crossing 阳维郄穴 Xi-cleft point of the yang linking vessel

Location: On the lateral aspect of the lower leg, 7 cun proximal to the tip of the external malleolus, on the posterior border of the fibula.

Acupuncture: Insert the needle perpendicularly to a depth of 1.0–1.5 cun and stimulate until there is a sore, numb sensation in the local area radiating to the foot.

Moxibustion: Apply 3–5 moxa cones or needle-warming moxibustion or, alternatively, hold a moxa stick above the point for 5–10 minutes.

Functions:

- Regulates gallbladder qi and calms the spirit
- Activates the channel and alleviates pain

Indications: Manic psychosis and epilepsy. Sore throat.

16 跗阳 (Fūyáng) BL 59 Supporting Yang 阳跷郄穴 Xi-cleft point of the yang motility vessel

Location: On the posterior aspect of the lower leg, posterior to the external malleolus, 3 cun superior to BL 60 (kūnlún).

Acupuncture: Insert the needle perpendicularly to a depth of 0.5–1.0 cun and stimulate until there is a sore, numb sensation in the local area radiating to the heel.

Moxibustion: Apply 3–5 moxa cones or needle-warming moxibustion or, alternatively, hold a moxa stick above the point for 5–10 minutes.

Functions:

- Activates the channel and alleviates pain
- Benefits the lumbar region and lower limbs
- Expels wind and clears heat

Indications: Pain in the lower back, sacrum, hip, lateral thigh and knee.

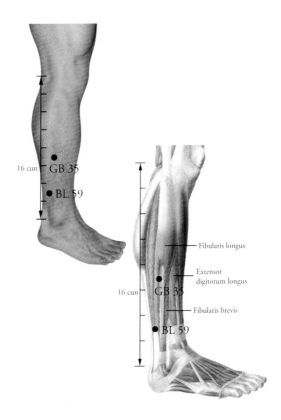

FIGURE 4.7

CHAPTER 5

Back-Shu Points

1 肺俞 (Fèishū) BL 13 Lung Shu 肺之背俞穴 Back-shu point of the lung

Location: On the upper back, 1.5 cun lateral to the lower border of the spinous process of the 3rd thoracic vertebra.

Acupuncture:

1. Insert the needle obliquely towards the spine to a depth of 0.5–0.8 cun and stimulate until there is a sore, numb sensation in the local area radiating to the intercostal space.

2. Avoid deep insertion to prevent pneumo-thorax.

Moxibustion: Apply 5–7 moxa cones or needle-warming moxibustion or, alternatively, hold a herbal moxa stick above the point for 10–20 minutes. Treat once a day, 20 days a month, to prevent common colds.

Functions:

- Tonifies lung qi and nourishes lung yin
- Descends and disperses lung qi
- Clears heat and releases the exterior

Indications: Cough, hemoptysis and sore throat. Palpitations. Pruritus, urticaria and acne. Back pain, night sweats and tidal fever.

2 厥阴俞 (Juéyīnshū) BL 14
Jueyin Shu 心包之背俞穴 Back-shu point of the pericardium

Location: On the upper back, 1.5 cun lateral to the lower border of the spinous process of the 4th thoracic vertebra.

Acupuncture:

1. Insert the needle obliquely towards the spine to a depth of 0.5–0.8 cun and stimulate until there is a sore, numb sensation in the local area radiating to the intercostal space.

2. Avoid deep insertion to prevent pneumothorax.

Moxibustion: Apply 5–9 moxa cones or needle-warming moxibustion or, alternatively, hold a moxa stick above the point for 10–20 minutes.

Functions:

- Spreads liver qi
- Relieves congestion in the chest and regulates qi

Indications: Cardiac pain and palpitations. Chest and hypochondrium distention and cough.

3 心俞 (Xīnshū) BL 15 Heart Shu
心之背俞穴 Back-shu
point of the heart

Location: On the upper back, 1.5 cun lateral to the lower border of the spinous process of the 5th thoracic vertebra.

Acupuncture:

1. Insert the needle obliquely towards the spine to a depth of 0.5–0.8 cun and stimulate until there is a sore, numb sensation in the local area radiating to the intercostal space.

2. Insert the needle subcutaneously either upwards or downwards to a depth of 1.0–2.0 cun and stimulate until there is a sore, numb sensation in the local area.

3. Avoid deep insertion to prevent pneumothorax.

Moxibustion: Apply 5–7 moxa cones or needle-warming moxibustion or, alternatively, hold a herbal moxa stick above the point for 10–20 minutes. Treat once a day, 20 days a month, to prevent common colds.

Functions:

• Tonifies and nourishes the heart

• Regulates heart qi and calms the spirit

• Relieves congestion in the chest and resolves blood stasis

• Clears heart fire

Indications: Cardiac pain, palpitations, chest distention and insomnia. Epilepsy and amnesia. Pain in the chest, shoulder and back.

4 肝俞 (Gānshū) BL 18
Liver Shu 肝之背俞穴 Back-shu point of the liver

Location: On the back, 1.5 cun lateral to the lower border of the spinous process of the 9th thoracic vertebra.

Acupuncture:

1. Insert the needle obliquely towards the spine to a depth of 0.5–0.8 cun and stimulate until there is a sore, numb sensation in the local area radiating to the intercostal space.

2. Insert the needle obliquely downwards to a depth of 1–1.5 cun and stimulate until there is a sore, numb sensation in the local area.

3. Avoid deep insertion to prevent pneumothorax.

Moxibustion: Apply 5–9 moxa cones or needle-warming moxibustion or, alternatively, hold a moxa stick above the point for 10–20 minutes.

Functions:

- Clears liver and gallbladder heat
- Spreads liver qi
- Regulates and nourishes liver blood
- Pacifies wind and calms the spirit
- Clears dampness and heat
- Benefits the eyes and sinews

Indications: Abdominal distention. Chest congestion. Epilepsy and dizziness. Headache, pain and redness of the eyes and blurred vision. Lumbago.

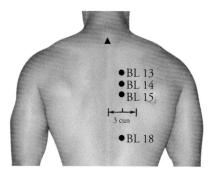

• BL 13
• BL 14
• BL 15

|← 3 cun →|

• BL 18

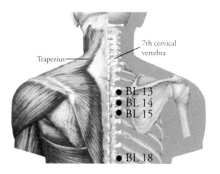

7th cervical vertebra

Trapezius

• BL 13
• BL 14
• BL 15

• BL 18

FIGURE 5.1

5 胆俞 (Dǎnshū) BL 19 Gallbladder Shu 胆之背俞穴 Back-shu point of the gallbladder

Location: On the back, 1.5 cun lateral to the lower border of the spinous process of the 10th thoracic vertebra.

Acupuncture:

1. Insert the needle obliquely towards the spine to a depth of 0.5–0.8 cun and stimulate until there is a sore, numb sensation in the local area radiating to the intercostal space.

2. Avoid deep insertion to prevent pneumothorax.

Moxibustion: Apply 5–9 moxa cones or needle-warming moxibustion or, alternatively, hold a herbal moxa stick above the point for 10–20 minutes. Treat once a day, 20 days a month.

Functions:

- Clears dampness and heat of the liver and gallbladder
- Clears heat and nourishes yin
- Clears pathogenic factors of shaoyang

- Harmonizes the stomach and descends qi
- Tonifies and regulates gallbladder

Indications: Abdominal distention, a poor appetite, vomiting of bile, a bitter taste in the mouth and hiccups. Yellow discoloration of the sclera.

6 脾俞 (Píshū) BL 20 Spleen Shu 脾之背俞穴 Back-shu point of the spleen

Location: On the back, 1.5 cun lateral to the lower border of the spinous process of the 11th thoracic vertebra.

Acupuncture:

1. Insert the needle obliquely towards the spine to a depth of 0.5–0.8 cun and stimulate until there is a sore, numb sensation in the local area radiating to the intercostal space.

2. Avoid deep insertion to prevent pneumothorax.

Moxibustion: Apply 5–9 moxa cones or needle-warming moxibustion or, alternatively, hold a herbal moxa stick above the point for 10–20 minutes. Treat once a day, 20 days a month, using 100 moxa cones in total.

Functions:

- Invigorates the spleen and benefits qi
- Tonifies spleen qi to control the blood
- Regulates and harmonizes the qi of the middle heater
- Resolves dampness

Indications: Abdominal distention, vomiting, diarrhea, dysentery, stomach ache, vomiting and blood in stools and urine. Lumbago.

7 胃俞 (Wèishū) BL 21 Stomach Shu 胃之背俞穴 Back-shu point of the stomach

Location: On the back, 1.5 cun lateral to the lower border of the spinous process of the 12th thoracic vertebra.

Acupuncture: Insert the needle perpendicularly to a depth of 0.5–0.8 cun and stimulate until there is a sore, numb sensation in the local area radiating to the abdomen.

Moxibustion: Apply 5–9 moxa cones or needle-warming moxibustion or, alternatively, hold a moxa stick above the point for 10–20 minutes.

Functions:

- Invigorates the spleen and harmonizes the stomach
- Resolves dampness and promotes digestion
- Harmonizes the middle heater

Indications: Pain in the chest and hypochondriac region. Epigastric pain, a poor appetite, abdominal distention, borborygmus, diarrhea, nausea and vomiting.

8 三焦俞 (Sānjiāoshū) BL 22 Three Heater Shu 三焦之背俞穴 Back-shu point of the three heater

Location: On the lower back, 1.5 cun lateral to the lower border of the spinous process of the 1st lumbar vertebra.

Acupuncture: Insert the needle perpendicularly to a depth of 0.5–0.8 cun and stimulate until there is a sore, numb sensation in the local area radiating to the abdomen.

Moxibustion: Apply 5–9 moxa cones or needle-warming moxibustion or, alternatively, hold a moxa stick above the point for 10–20 minutes.

Functions:

- Regulates the three heater and resolves dampness
- Regulates the fluid passages and promotes urination
- Benefits original qi
- Tonifies the lumbar region and knees

Indications: Edema, dysuria and enuresis. Vomiting, hiccupping, undigested food, borborygmus, diarrhea and lumbago.

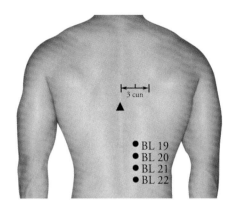

3 cun

▲

● BL 19
● BL 20
● BL 21
● BL 22

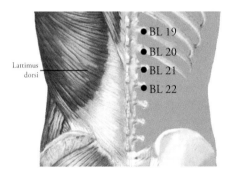

Lattimus
dorsi

● BL 19

● BL 20

● BL 21

● BL 22

FIGURE 5.2

9 肾俞 (Shènshū) BL 23
Kidney Shu 肾之背俞穴 Back-shu point of the kidney

Location: On the lower back, 1.5 cun lateral to the lower border of the spinous process of the 2nd lumbar vertebra.

Acupuncture: Insert the needle perpendicularly to a depth of 0.5–0.8 cun and stimulate until there is a sore, numb sensation in the local area radiating to the hip and down the leg.

Moxibustion: Apply 5–9 moxa cones or needle-warming moxibustion or, alternatively, hold a herbal moxa stick above the point for 10–20 minutes.

Functions:

- Tonifies kidney and fortifies yang
- Benefits original qi
- Nourishes kidney yin
- Strenthens kidney qi and the lumbar region
- Regulates the fluid passages and benefits urination
- Benefits the ears and eyes

Indications: Spermatorrhea, enuresis, edema, dysuria and impotence, Irregular menstruation, morbid leucorrhea and infertility. Blurred vision, tinnitus and deafness. Pain and soreness of the lower back and knees.

10 大肠俞 (Dàchángshū) BL 25
Large Intestine Shu 大肠之背俞穴
Back-shu point of the large intestine

Location: On the lower back, 1.5 cun lateral to the lower border of the spinous process of the 4th lumbar vertebra.

Acupuncture:

1. Insert the needle perpendicularly to a depth of 0.5–0.8 cun and stimulate until there is a sore, numb sensation in the local area radiating to the hip and down the leg.

2. Insert the needle subcutaneously towards BL 27 (xiǎochángshù) to a depth of 2.0–2.5 cun and stimulate until there is a sore, numb sensation in the local area.

3. Insert the needle obliquely to a depth of 2.0–2.5 cun and stimulate until there

is an electric sensation in the local area radiating to the hip and down the leg.

Moxibustion: Apply 5–9 moxa cones or needle-warming moxibustion or, alternatively, hold a herbal moxa stick above the point for 10–20 minutes.

Functions:

- Regulates the intestines and stomach
- Regulates qi and removes stagnation
- Tonifies the lumbar region and lower limbs

Indications: Abdominal pain and distention, diarrhea, borborygmus, constipation and dysentery. Lumbago.

11 小肠俞 (Xiǎochángshū) BL 27 Small Intestine Shu 小肠之背俞穴 Back-shu point of the small intestine

Location: On the lower back, 1.5 cun lateral to the lower border of the spinous process of the 1st sacral vertebra.

Acupuncture:

1. Insert the needle perpendicularly to a depth of 0.8–1.0 cun and stimulate until there is a sore, numb sensation in the local area.

2. Insert the needle obliquely towards the spine to a depth of 2.0–2.5 cun and stimulate until there is a sore, numb sensation in the local area.

Moxibustion: Apply 5–9 moxa cones or needle-warming moxibustion or, alternatively, hold a moxa stick above the point for 10–20 minutes.

Functions:

- Clears heat and resolves dampness
- Separates the pure and the turbid
- Regulates the intestines and bladder
- Regulates small intestine qi

Indications: Dysentery, diarrhea, distention and pain in the lower abdomen, hernia and hemorrhoids. Spermatorrhea, enuresis and blood in urine. Morbid leucorrhea. Weakness and pain of the lower back and knees.

12 膀胱俞 (Pángguāngshū) BL 28
Bladder Shu 膀胱之背俞穴
Back-shu point of the bladder

Location: On the sacrum, 1.5 cun lateral to the middle of the sacral crest, on a level with the 2nd posterior sacral foramen.

Acupuncture: Insert the needle perpendicularly to a depth of 0.5–0.8 cun and stimulate until there is a sore, numb sensation in the local area.

Moxibustion: Apply 5–9 moxa cones or needle-warming moxibustion or, alternatively, hold a moxa stick above the point for 10–20 minutes.

Functions:

- Tonifies original qi and benefits essence
- Benefits the lumbar region and lower limbs

- Clears dampness and heat in the lower heater
- Regulates the bladder

Indications: Difficulty and redness of urination, hesitancy and obstruction, enuresis and spermatorrhea. Abdominal pain, diarrhea and constipation. Stiffness and pain in the waist and spine.

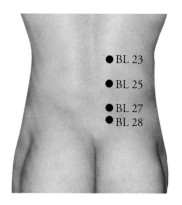

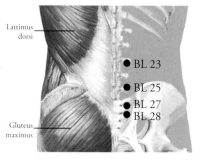

FIGURE 5.3

CHAPTER 6

Front-Mu Points

1 中府 (Zhóngfǔ) LU 1
Central Palace 肺募穴 Front-mu point of the lung

Location: On the lateral aspect of the chest, 1 cun inferior to LU 2 (yúnmén), in the 1st intercostal space and lateral to the front midline.

Acupuncture:

1. Insert the needle perpendicularly to a depth of 0.3–0.5 cun and stimulate the needle until there is a sore sensation in the local area radiating to the chest or the arms.

2. Insert the needle obliquely outward to a depth of 0.5–0.8 cun and stimulate the needle until there is a sensation in the local area.

Moxibustion: Apply 3–5 moxa cones or warm-needle moxibustion or, alternatively, hold a moxa stick above the point for 10–20 minutes to keep the local area warm and comfortable. Apply moxibustion once a day for 20 days every month to promote general health and well-being.

Functions:

- Disperses and descends lung qi and clears heat
- Alleviates cough and wheezing
- Transforms phlegm
- Regulates the fluid passageways
- Tonifies qi and invigorates the spleen

Indications: Cough, asthma and chest pain. Shoulder pain, upper back pain, diseases of the shoulder joint.

2 巨阙 (Jùquè) CV 14 Great Gate
心募穴 Front-mu point of the heart

Location: On the upper abdomen, on the anterior midline, 2 cun inferior to the sternocostal angle.

Acupuncture:

1. Insert the needle perpendicularly to a depth of 0.5–1.0 cun and stimulate until there is a sore, distending sensation in the local area radiating to the upper abdomen.

2. Insert the needle obliquely either downwards or upwards to a depth of 4.0–5.0 cun stimulate until there is a sore, distending sensation in the local area to treat vomiting.

3. Acupuncture is prohibited in hepatomegaly or splenomegaly.

Moxibustion: Apply 5–7 moxa cones or needle-warming moxibustion or, alternatively, hold a moxa stick above the point for 10–20 minutes.

Functions:

- Transforms phlegm and calms the spirit
- Descends lung qi and relieves congestion in the chest
- Regulates qi and alleviates pain
- Harmonizes the stomach and descends rebellious qi

Indications: Disorders of the heart: pain of the chest and cardiac pain.

3 膻中 (Dánzhōng) CV 17 Chest Center 心包募穴 Front-mu point of the pericardium

Location: On the chest, on the anterior midline, at the level of the 4th intercostal space, at the midpoint between the two nipples.

Acupuncture: Insert the needle subcutaneously or obliquely to a depth of 0.3–0.5 cun and stimulate until there is a sore, distending sensation in the local area radiating to the chest.

Moxibustion: Apply 5–9 moxa cones or needle-warming moxibustion or, alternatively, hold a moxa stick above the point for 10–20 minutes.

Functions:

- Relieves congestion in the chest and regulates qi
- Descends rebellious qi of the lung and stomach
- Alleviates cough and wheezing
- Benefits the breasts and promotes lactation

Indications: Infantile milk regurgitation. Chest distention, cough and insufficient lactation. Heart palpitations, irritability and cardiac pain.

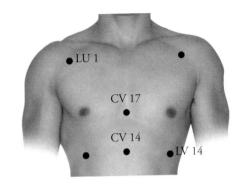

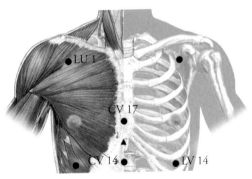

Figure 6.1

4 中脘 (Zhōngwǎn) CV 12 Middle Venter 胃募穴 Front-mu points of the stomach

Location: On the upper abdomen, on the anterior midline, 4 cun superior to the umbilicus.

Acupuncture: Insert the needle perpendicularly to a depth of 0.5–1.0 cun and stimulate until there is a sore, distending sensation in the local area.

Moxibustion: Apply 5–9 moxa cones or needle-warming moxibustion or, alternatively, hold a moxa stick above the point for 15–20 minutes. Apply indirect moxibustion 3–5 times a day, 20 days a month to promote general good health and well-being.

Functions:

- Invigorates the spleen and harmonizes the stomach
- Warms the middle heater and descends rebellious qi
- Regulates qi and alleviates pain

Indications: Stomach ache, abdominal distention, borborygmus and abdominal pain. Irregular menstruation, dysmenorrhea, amenorrhea and metrorrhagia.

5 日月 (Rìyuè) GB 24 Sun and Moon 胆募穴 Front-mu point of gallbladder

Location: On the upper abdomen, directly below the nipple, in the 7th intercostal space, 4 cun lateral to the anterior midline.

Acupuncture: Insert the needle subcutaneously to a depth of 0.5–0.8 cun and stimulate until there is a sore, numb sensation in the local area radiating to the chest and hypochondrium.

Moxibustion: Apply 3–5 indirect moxa or hold a moxa stick above the point for 5–10 minutes.

Functions:

- Lowers rebellious qi and benefits the gallbladder
- Spreads liver qi and resolves dampness and heat
- Harmonizes the intestine and stomach

Indications: Vomiting and stomach ache. Jaundice. Chest distention and pain of the hypochondrium.

6 期门 (Qīmén) LV 14 Period Door
肝募穴 Front-mu point of the liver

Location: On the chest, directly inferior to the nipple, in the 6th intercostal space, 4 cun lateral to the anterior midline.

Acupuncture: Insert the needle obliquely or along the intercostal space 0.5–1.0 cun and stimulate until there is a sore, numb sensation in the local area radiating to the back.

Moxibustion: Apply 5–9 moxa cones or needle-warming moxibustion or, alternatively, hold a moxa stick above the point for 10–20 minutes.

Functions:

- Spreads liver qi and regulates qi
- Harmonizes the liver and stomach

Indications: Distention of the chest and hypochondrium, cough and asthma.

7 天枢 (Tiānshū) ST 25 Celestial Pivot 大肠募穴 Front-mu point of the large intestine

Location: On the abdomen, 2 cun lateral to the umbilicus.

Acupuncture:

1. Insert the needle perpendicularly to a depth of 1.0–1.5 cun and stimulate until there is a sore, numb sensation in the local area radiating to the side of the abdomen.

2. Insert the needle slightly obliquely and stimulate until there is a sensation radiating to the abdomen reaching ST 19 (bùróng).

3. Insert the needle slightly obliquely towards ST 28 (shuǐdào) and stimulate until there is a sensation radiating to ST 29 (guīlái).

Moxibustion: Apply 5–10 moxa cones or needle-warming moxibustion or, alternatively, hold a moxa stick above the point for 15–30 minutes.

Apply moxibustion once a day, 20 times every month, until the skin feels warm and comfortable or until the local area becomes slightly red to enhance general health and well-being.

Functions:

- Invigorates the spleen and stomach
- Regulates the spleen and stomach
- Regulates the intestines
- Resolves dampness and damp-heat
- Regulates qi and eliminates stagnation

Indications: Vomiting, hematemesis, abdominal distention, borborygmus, pain around the umbilicus, dysentery, constipation and hernia. Irregular menstruation, dysmenorrhea, amenorrhea and metrorrhagia. Epilepsy, headache and insomnia with copious dreams. Dysuria and lumbago. Dizziness and urticaria.

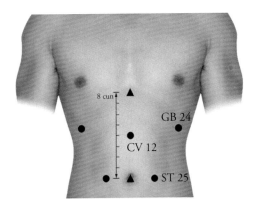

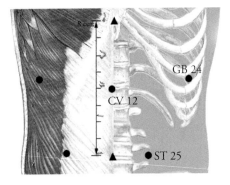

FIGURE 6.2

8 石门 (Shímén) CV 5 Stone Gate 三焦募穴 Front-mu point of the three heater

Location: On the lower abdomen, on the anterior midline, 2 cun inferior to the umbilicus.

Acupuncture: Insert the needle perpendicularly to a depth of 0.5–1.0 cun and stimulate until there is a sore, distending sensation in the local area radiating to the genitalia.

Moxibustion: Apply 5–9 moxa cones or hold a moxa stick above the point for 10–20 minutes.

Functions:

- Invigorates the spleen and tonifies the kidney
- Clears the lower heater
- Benefits the water passages
- Regulates qi and alleviates pain
- Regulates the uterus

Indications: Spermatorrhea, impotence and enuresis. Irregular menstruation, dysmenorrhea and morbid leucorrhea.

9 关元 (Guānyuán) CV 4
Origin Pass 小肠募穴 Front-mu point of the small intestine

Location: On the lower abdomen, on the anterior midline, 3 cun inferior to the umbilicus.

Acupuncture: Insert the needle perpendicularly to a depth of 0.5–1.0 cun and stimulate until there is a sore, distending sensation in the local area radiating to the genitalia.

Moxibustion: Apply 5–9 moxa cones or hold a moxa stick above the point for 10–20 minutes.

Functions:

- Tonifies original qi and benefits essence
- Tonifies deficiencies
- Tonifies and nourishes the kidney
- Regulates menstruation and leucorrhea
- Benefits the uterus and assists conception
- Regulates the small intestine
- Regulates the penetrating and conception vessels

Indications: Irregular menstruation, dysmenorrhea and morbid leucorrhea. Spermatorrhea, impotence and enuresis. Stroke. General weakness.

10 中极 (Zhōngjí) CV 3
Central Pivot 膀胱募穴 Front-mu point of the bladder

Location: On the lower abdomen, on the anterior midline, 4 cun inferior to the umbilicus.

Acupuncture:

1. Insert the needle perpendicularly to a depth of 0.5–1.0 cun and stimulate until there is a sore, distending sensation in the local area radiating to the genitalia.

2. Request that the patient empties their bladder before needling this point.

Moxibustion: Apply 3–5 moxa cones or hold a moxa stick above the point for 5–15 minutes. Moxibustion is prohibited during pregnancy.

Functions:

- Transforms dampness and clears heat
- Treats leucorrhea

- Benefits the uterus and regulates menstruation
- Dispels stagnation and benefits the lower heater
- Tonifies the kidney and benefits the bladder

Indications: Spermatorrhea, impotence and enuresis. Irregular menstruation, dysmenorrhea and morbid leucorrhea.

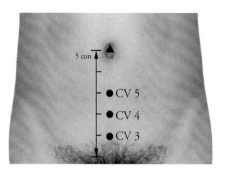

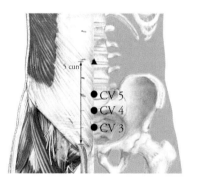

FIGURE 6.3

11 章门 (Zhāngmén) LV 13 Veil Door
脾募穴 Front-mu point of the spleen

Location: On the lateral aspect of the abdomen, below the free end of the 11th floating rib.

Acupuncture:

1. Insert the needle obliquely to a depth of 0.5–0.8 cun and stimulate until there is a sore, numb sensation in the local area radiating to the external genitalia.

2. Avoid deep insertion to prevent puncturing the liver or spleen.

Moxibustion: Apply 5–9 moxa cones or needle-warming moxibustion or, alternatively, hold a moxa stick above the point for 10–20 minutes.

Functions:

- Spreads liver qi and regulates qi
- Harmonizes the liver and spleen
- Invigorates the spleen and tonifies qi

- Descends rebellious qi and regulates the stomach

Indications: Abdominal congestion and pain, borborygmus, vomiting, edema, jaundice diarrhea and constipation.

12 京门 (Jīngmén) GB 25
Capital Door 肾募穴 Front-mu point of the kidney

Location: On the lateral aspect of the abdomen, 1.8 cun posterior to LV 13 (zhǎngmén), on the lower border of the end of the 12th floating rib.

Acupuncture: Insert the needle subcutaneously to a depth of 0.5–0.8 cun and stimulate until there is a sore, numb sensation in the local area radiating to the lower back.

Moxibustion: Apply 5–9 moxa cones or hold a moxa stick above the point for 10–20 minutes.

Functions:

- Tonifies the kidney and benefits the lumbar region
- Regulates fluid passages
- Invigorates the spleen and regulates the intestines

Indications: Hiccups, stomach ache and acid regurgitation. Chest distention and pain in the hypochondrium.

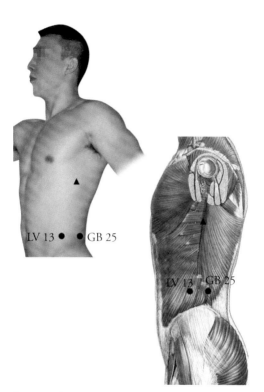

FIGURE 6.4

CHAPTER 7

Lower He-Sea Points

1 上巨虛 (Shàngjùxū) ST 37 Upper Great Void 大肠下合穴 Lower he-sea point of large intestine

Location: On the anterior, lateral aspect of the leg, 3 cun distal to ST 36 (zúsānlǐ), one finger's breadth lateral to the anterior ridge of the tibia.

Acupuncture:

1. Insert the needle perpendicularly to a depth of 1.0–2.0 cun and stimulate until there is a sore, numb sensation in the local area radiating upwards or downwards.

2. Insert the needle slightly obliquely and stimulate until there is a sensation radiating to the knees and abdomen, and in some cases the sensation can radiate to the upper abdomen and chest area.

3. Insert the needle slightly obliquely downwards and stimulate until the sensation radiates to the dorsum of the foot and toes.

Moxibustion: Apply 5–9 moxa cones or needle-warming moxibustion or, alternatively, hold a moxa stick above the point for 10–20 minutes.

Functions:

- Regulates the spleen and stomach
- Activates the channel and alleviates pain
- Regulates the intestines and transforms stagnation
- Clears damp heat and alleviates diarrhea

Indications: Dyspepsia, dysentery, diarrhea, constipation, abdominal distention and borborygmus.

2 下巨虚 (Xiàjùxū) ST 39 Lower Great Void 小肠下合穴 Lower he-sea point of the small intestine

Location: On the anterior and lateral aspect of the leg, 9 cun distal to ST 35 (dúbí), one finger's breadth lateral to the anterior ridge of the tibia.

Acupuncture: Insert the needle perpendicularly to a depth of 1.0–2.0 cun and stimulate until there is a sore, numb sensation in the local area which radiates to the dorsum of the foot.

Moxibustion: Apply 5–9 moxa cones or needle-warming moxibustion or, alternatively, hold a moxa stick above the point for 10–20 minutes.

Functions:

- Regulates small intestine qi and transforms stagnation
- Harmonizes the intestines and clears damp-heat
- Activates the channel and alleviates pain

Indications: Abdominal distention and borborygmus. A low appetite, abdominal pain and dysentery.

3 足三里 (Zúsānlǐ) ST 36 Three Leg Miles 胃下合穴 Lower he-sea point of the stomach

Location: On the anterior aspect of the lower leg, 3 cun distal to ST 35 (dúbí), one finger's breadth lateral from the anterior ridge of the tibia.

Acupuncture:

1. Insert the needle perpendicularly to a depth of 0.5–1.5 cun and stimulate until there is a sensation radiating to the ankle and dorsum of the foot and toes.

2. Insert the needle obliquely upwards and stimulate until there is a sensation radiating to ST 31 (bìguān), ST 29 (guīlái) and ST 25 (tiānshū).

Moxibustion: Apply 5–10 moxa cones or needle-warming moxibustion or, alternatively, hold a moxa stick over the point for 10–20 minutes. Apply scarring moxibustion once a year or apply 5–10 moxa cones once a day, 20 days a month to promote general health and well-being.

Functions:

- Invigorates the spleen and harmonizes the stomach
- Supports correct qi and nourishes original qi
- Activates the channel and alleviates pain
- Regulates qi and resolves dampness
- Tonifies qi and nourishes blood
- Prevents disease and benefits macrobiosis

Indications: Stomach ache, vomiting, abdominal distention, borborygmus, indigestion, diarrhea, constipation and dysentery. Epilepsy and stroke. Wheezing with phlegm, carbuncle weakness and hemoptysis. Dysuria, enuresis and hernia. Palpitations. Gynecological disorders such as eclampsia, bloody and excessive leucorrhea, dysmenorrhea, postnatal lumbago. Pain in the knees and shins, paralysis of the lower limbs, sciatica and conditions of the knee and local area. Insomnia.

4 阳陵泉 (Yánglíngquán) GB 34 Yang Mound Spring 胆下合穴 Lower he-sea point of the gallbladder

Location: In a sitting position with the knee bent at 90° or in the supine position, the point is located in a depression anterior and inferior to the head of the fibula.

Acupuncture:

1. Insert the needle perpendicularly towards SP 9 (yīnlíngquán) to a depth of 1.0–3.0 cun and stimulate until there is a sore, numb sensation in the local area radiating downwards.

2. Insert the needle obliquely 0.5–0.8 cun and stimulate until there is a sore, numb sensation in the local area.

Moxibustion: Apply 3–5 moxa cones or needle-warming moxibustion or, alternatively, hold a moxa stick above the point for 5–10 minutes.

Functions:

- Relaxes sinews and benefits the joints
- Activates the channel and alleviates pain
- Spreads liver and gallbladder qi
- Clears liver and gallbladder dampness and heat

Indications: Headache, tinnitus, deafness and eye pain. Asthma and cough. Incontinence and enuresis. Pain in the chest, hypochondrium and knees, weakness and numbness of the lower extremities and hemiplegia.

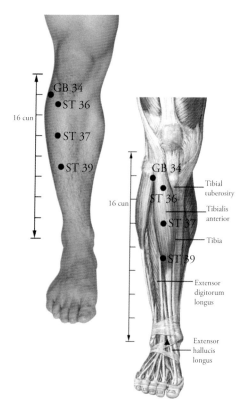

FIGURE 7.1

5 委中 (Wěizhōng) BL 40 Bend Middle 膀胱下合穴 Lower he-sea point of the bladder

Location: At the midpoint of the transverse crease of the popliteal fossa, between the tendons of the muscles biceps femoris and semitendinous.

Acupuncture:

1. Insert the needle perpendicularly to a depth of 0.5–1.0 cun and stimulate until there is a sore, distending and numb sensation radiating to the calf and foot.

2. Prick with a three-edged needle to bleed.

Moxibustion: Apply 3–5 moxa cones or needle-warming moxibustion or, alternatively, hold a moxa stick above the point for 10–20 minutes.

Functions:

- Benefits the lumbar region and knees
- Activates the channel and alleviates pain
- Cools the blood and clears summer heat
- Stops vomiting and diarrhea

Indications: Lumbar pain, joint pain due to stagnation of damp-cold and hemiplegia. Erysipelas, boils, furuncle, bruises and spontaneous bleeding under the skin. Abdominal pain, vomiting and diarrhea.

6 委阳 (Wěiyáng) BL 39 Yang Bend 三焦下合穴 Lower he-sea point of the three heater

Location: At the lateral end of the popliteal transverse crease, on the medial side of the tendon of the muscle biceps femoris.

Acupuncture: Insert the needle perpendicularly to a depth of 0.5–1.0 cun and stimulate until there is a sore, numb sensation radiating to the calf and foot.

Moxibustion: Apply 3–5 moxa cones or needle-warming moxibustion or, alternatively, hold a moxa stick above the point for 10–20 minutes.

Functions:

- Regulates the three heater
- Regulates urination
- Activates the channel and alleviates pain

Indications: Urinal dribbling. Constipation. Pain in the back and lumbar region.

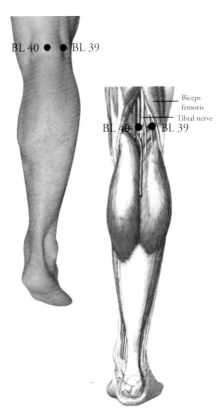

FIGURE 7.2

CHAPTER 8

Eight Influence Points

1 章门 (Zhāngmén) LV 13
Veil Door 脏会 Influence
point of the zang organs

Location: On the lateral aspect of the abdomen, below the free end of the 11th floating rib.

Acupuncture:

1. Insert the needle obliquely to a depth of 0.5–0.8 cun and stimulate until there is a sore, numb sensation in the local area radiating to the external genitalia.

2. Avoid deep insertion to prevent puncturing the liver or spleen.

Moxibustion: Apply 5–9 moxa cones or needle-warming moxibustion or, alternatively, hold a moxa stick above the point for 10–20 minutes.

Functions:

• Spreads liver qi and regulates qi

- Harmonizes the liver and spleen
- Invigorates the spleen and tonifies qi
- Descends rebellious qi and regulates the stomach

Indications: Abdominal congestion and pain, borborygmus, vomiting, edema, jaundice, diarrhea and constipation.

2 中脘 (Zhōngwǎn) CV 12 Central Stomach 腑会 Influence point of the fu organs

Location: On the upper abdomen, on the anterior midline, 4 cun superior to the umbilicus.

Acupuncture: Insert the needle perpendicularly to a depth of 0.5–1.0 cun and stimulate until there is a sore, distending sensation in the local area.

Moxibustion: Apply 5–9 moxa cones or needle-warming moxibustion or, alternatively, hold a moxa stick above the point for 15–20 minutes. Apply indirect moxibustion 3–5 times a day, 20 days a month, to promote general good health and well-being.

Functions:

- Invigorates the spleen and harmonizes the stomach
- Warms the middle heater and descends rebellious qi
- Regulates qi and alleviates pain

Indications: Stomach ache, abdominal distention, borborygmus and abdominal pain. Irregular menstruation, dysmenorrhea, amenorrhea and metrorrhagia.

3 膻中 (Dánzhōng) CV 17 Chest Center 气会 Influence point of qi

Location: On the chest, on the anterior midline, at the level of the 4th intercostal space, at the midpoint between the two nipples.

Acupuncture: Insert the needle subcutaneously or obliquely to a depth of 0.3–0.5 cun and stimulate until there is a sore, distending sensation in the local area radiating to the chest.

Moxibustion: Apply 5–9 moxa cones or needle-warming moxibustion or, alternatively, hold a moxa stick above the point for 10–20 minutes.

Functions:

- Relieves congestion in the chest and regulates qi
- Descends rebellious qi of the lung and stomach
- Alleviates cough and wheezing
- Benefits the breasts and promotes lactation

Indications: Infantile milk regurgitation. Chest distention, cough and insufficient lactation. Heart palpitations, irritability and cardiac pain.

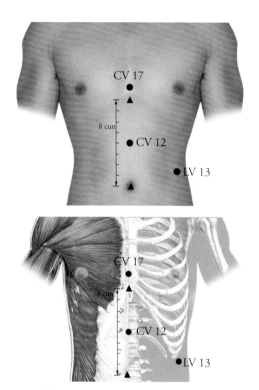

Figure 8.1

4 膈俞 (Géshū) BL 17 Diaphragm Shu 血会 Influence point of the blood

Location: On the back, 1.5 cun lateral to the lower border of the spinous process of the 7th thoracic vertebra.

Acupuncture: Insert the needle subcutaneously or obliquely to a depth of 0.3–0.5 cun and stimulate until there is a sore, distending sensation in the local area radiating to the chest.

Moxibustion: Apply 5–9 moxa cones or needle-warming moxibustion or, alternatively, hold a moxa stick above the point for 10–20 minutes.

Functions:

- Relieves congestion in the chest and regulates qi
- Descends rebellious qi of the lung and stomach
- Alleviates cough and wheezing
- Benefits the breasts and promotes lactation

Indications: Cardiac pain, palpitations and anemia. Vomiting, hiccupping, abdominal pain, hemoptysis and blood in the stools. Asthma, coughing, sore throat and chest congestion with excessive phlegm. Back ache. Night sweating.

5 大杼 (Dàzhù) BL 11 Great Pillar
骨会 Influence point of the bone

Location: On the upper back, 1.5 cun lateral to the lower border of the spinous process of the 1st thoracic vertebra.

Acupuncture: Insert the needle subcutaneously or obliquely to a depth of 0.3–0.5 cun and stimulate until there is a sore, distending sensation in the local area radiating to the chest.

Moxibustion: Apply 5–9 moxa cones or needle-warming moxibustion or, alternatively, hold a moxa stick above the point for 10–20 minutes.

Functions:

- Relieves congestion in the chest and regulates qi
- Descends rebellious qi of the lung and stomach
- Alleviates cough and wheezing
- Benefits the breasts and promotes lactation

Indications: Neck stiffness, headache, pain in the shoulder and back. Cough and nasal obstruction. Dizziness.

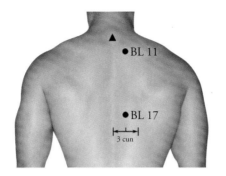

BL 11

BL 17

3 cun

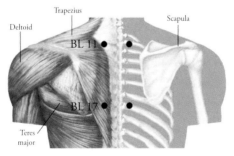

Trapezius

Scapula

Deltoid

BL 11

BL 17

Teres
major

FIGURE 8.2

6 悬钟 (Xuánzhōng) GB 39
Suspended Bell 髓会 Influence point of the marrow

Location: On the lateral aspect of the lower leg, 3 cun proximal to the tip of the external malleolus, in the depression between the posterior border of the fibula and the muscles of peroneus longus and peroneus brevis.

Acupuncture: Insert the needle subcutaneously or obliquely to a depth of 0.3–0.5 cun and stimulate until there is a sore, distending sensation in the local area radiating to the chest.

Moxibustion: Apply 5–9 moxa cones or needle-warming moxibustion or, alternatively, hold a moxa stick above the point for 10–20 minutes.

Functions:

- Relieves congestions in the chest and regulates qi
- Descends rebellious qi of the lung and stomach
- Alleviates cough and wheezing
- Benefits the breasts and promotes lactation

Indications: Neck stiffness, pain of the chest and hypochondrium, swelling and pain in the axillary region, hemiplegia and pain of the heel. Abdominal distention. Dizziness. Tinnitus and deafness. High blood pressure.

7 阳陵泉 (Yánglíngquán)
GB 34 Yang Mound Spring 筋会
Influence point of the sinews

Location: In the sitting position with the knee bent at 90° or in the supine position, the point is located in the depression anterior and inferior to the head of the fibula.

Acupuncture:

1. Insert the needle perpendicularly towards SP 9 (yīnlíngquán) 1.0–3.0 cun and stimulate until there is a sore, numb sensation in the local area radiating downwards.

2. Insert the needle obliquely to a depth of 0.5–0.8 cun and stimulate until there is a sore, numb sensation in the local area.

Moxibustion: Apply 3–5 moxa cones or needle-warming moxibustion or, alternatively, hold a moxa stick above the point for 5–10 minutes.

Functions:

- Relaxes sinews and benefits the joints
- Activates the channel and alleviates pain
- Spreads liver and gallbladder qi
- Clears liver and gallbladder dampness and heat

Indications: Headache, tinnitus, deafness and eye pain. Asthma and coughing. Incontinence and enuresis. Pain in the chest, hypochondrium and knee, weakness and numbness of the lower extremities and hemiplegia.

8 太渊 (Tàiyuān) LU 9 Supreme Abyss 脉会 Influence point of the vessels

Location: On the transverse wrist crease, on the radial side of the radial artery where the radial pulse is palpable.

Acupuncture:

1. Insert the needle perpendicularly to a depth of 0.2–0.3 cun and stimulate until there is a numb, distending sensation in the local area.

2. Avoid puncturing the radial artery.

Moxibustion: Apply 1–3 moxa cones or hold a moxa stick above the point for 5–10 minutes. Scarring moxibustion is not applicable since the radial artery is located nearby.

Functions:

- Alleviates coughing and transforms phlegm
- Descends lung qi
- Regulates and harmonizes the vessels
- Activates the channel and alleviates pain
- Tonifies qi and invigorates the spleen

Indications: Pain in the wrist and pulseless disease (Takayasu's arteritis).

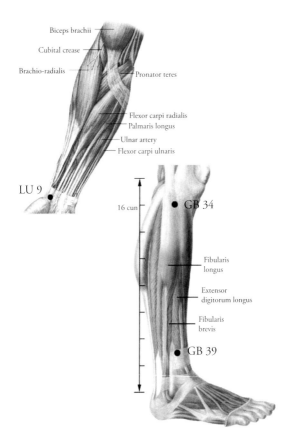

Biceps brachii

Cubital crease

Brachio-radialis

Pronator teres

Flexor carpi radialis

Palmaris longus

Ulnar artery

Flexor carpi ulnaris

LU 9

16 cun

GB 34

Fibularis longus

Extensor digitorum longus

Fibularis brevis

GB 39

FIGURE 8.3

CHAPTER 9

Eight Confluence Points

1 内关 (Nèiguān) PC 6 Inner Gate
八脉交会穴通阴维 Confluence point of the yang linking vessel

Location: On the palmar aspect of the forearm, 2 cun proximal to the transverse crease of the wrist, on the line connecting PC 3 (qūzé) to PC 7 (dàling).

Acupuncture: Insert the needle perpendicularly to a depth of 0.3–0.5 cun and stimulate until there is a sore, numb sensation in the local area radiating down the heart channel and reaching the ring or little finger, or reaching the head and chest.

Moxibustion: Apply 1–3 moxa cones or hold a moxa stick above the point for 10–20 minutes.

Functions:

- Calms the spirit
- Activates the channel and alleviates pain
- Benefits the throat and tongue

Indications: Cardiac pain, palpitations and insomnia. Chest distention and asthma. Stomach ache, vomiting and hiccupping.

2 列缺 (Lièquē) LU 7 Broken Sequence 八脉交会穴通 任脉 Confluence points of the conception vessel

Location: On the radial side of the forearm, 1.5 cun proximal to the transverse crease of the wrist, superior to the styloid process of the radius and between tendons of the muscles brachioradialis and abductor pollicis longus.

Acupuncture:

1. Insert the needle obliquely upward to a depth of 0.2–0.3 cun and stimulate until there is a sore, heavy and numb sensation in the local area radiating to the elbow and the shoulder.

2. Insert the needle obliquely downward to a depth of 0.3–0.5 cun and stimulate until there is a sensation in the local area.

Moxibustion: Apply 3–5 moxa cones or hold a moxa stick above the point for 5–10 minutes. Scarring moxibustion is not applicable since the skin is very thin at this point.

Functions:

- Releases the exterior and expels wind
- Regulates the conception vessel
- Regulates the fluid passageways
- Activates the channel and alleviates pain
- Promotes the descending functions of the lung
- Benefits the head and nape

Indications: Cough, sore throat, asthma and shortness of breath. Headache, migraine and neck stiffness.

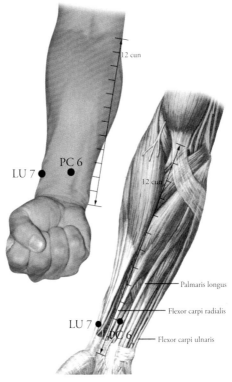

12 cun

LU 7 ● ● PC 6

12 cun

LU 7 ● ● PC 6

Palmaris longus

Flexor carpi radialis

Flexor carpi ulnaris

FIGURE 9.1

3 外关 (Wàiguān) TH 5 Outer Gate
八脉交会穴通阳维 Confluence points of the yang linking vessel

Location: On the dorsal aspect of the forearm, on the line connecting TH 4 (yangchí) to the tip of the elbow, 2 cun proximal to the transverse crease of the wrist, in the depression between the ulna and radius.

Acupuncture:

1. Insert the needle perpendicularly to a depth of 0.5–1.0 cun and stimulate until there is a sore, numb sensation in the local area radiating to the tip of the finger.

2. Insert the needle obliquely to a depth of 1.5–2.0 cun and stimulate until there is a sore, numb sensation in the local area radiating to the elbow and shoulder.

Moxibustion: Apply 3–5 moxa cones or needle-warming moxibustion or, alternatively, hold a moxa stick above the point for 3–5 minutes.

Functions:

- Expels wind, clears heat and releases the exterior
- Opens the yang linking vessel
- Activates the channel and alleviates pain

Indications: Headache, tinnitus, tooth ache and redness, swelling and pain in the eyes. Pain in the upper extremities. Febrile diseases.

4 后溪 (Hòuxī) SI 3 Posterior Valley
八脉交会穴通督脉 Confluence points of the governing vessel

Location: On the ulnar side of the hand, proximal to the 5th metacarpophalangeal joint, at the end of the transverse crease, at the junction where the skin changes texture.

Acupuncture: Insert the needle perpendicularly to a depth of 0.5–0.8 cun and stimulate until there is a sore, numb sensation in the local area spreading to the palm.

Moxibustion: Apply 1–3 moxa cones or hold a moxa stick above the point for 5–10 minutes.

Functions:

- Activates the channel and alleviates pain
- Clears wind and heat
- Calms the spirit and treats epilepsy
- Regulates the governing vessel
- Benefits the occiput, neck and back
- Revives consciousness

Indications: Tinnitus and deafness. Manic psychosis, epilepsy and stroke. Pain and rigidity of the head and neck. Febrile conditions, jaundice and malaria.

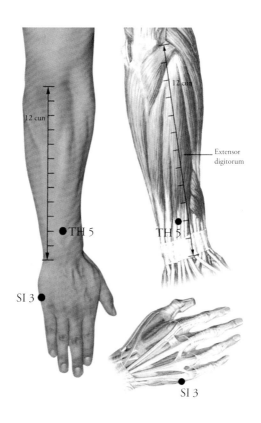

FIGURE 9.2

5 申脉 (Shēnmài) BL 62
Extended Vessel 八脉交会穴
通阳跷 Confluence points of
the yang motility vessel

Location: On the lateral side of the foot, in the depression directly inferior to the external malleolus.

Acupuncture: Insert the needle perpendicularly to a depth of 0.2–0.3 cun and stimulate until there is a sore, numb sensation in the local area.

Moxibustion: Apply 3–5 moxa cones or needle-warming moxibustion or, alternatively, hold a moxa stick above the point for 5–10 minutes.

Functions:

- Activates channel and alleviates pain
- Regulates the yang motility vessel
- Calms the heart and spirit
- Treats epilepsy

Indications: Insomnia, manic psychosis, epilepsy, stroke and unconsciousness. Headache and redness, swelling and pain of the eyes. Upper and lower back pain.

6 公孙 (Gōngsūn) SP 4
Yellow Emperor 八脉交会 穴通冲脉 Confluence point of the penetrating vessel

Location: On the medial side of the foot, in the depression anterior and inferior to the base of the 1st metatarsal bone, at the junction where the skin changes texture.

Acupuncture: Insert the needle perpendicularly towards KI 1 (yǒngquán) to a depth of 0.5–0.8 cun and stimulate until there is a sore numb sensation in the local area radiating to the sole of the foot.

Moxibustion: Apply 3–5 moxa cones or needle-warming moxibustion or, alternatively, hold a moxa stick above the point for 10–20 minutes.

Functions:

- Invigorates the spleen and harmonizes the middle heater
- Regulates qi and resolves dampness
- Regulates the penetrating and conception vessels
- Regulates qi

Indications: Vomiting, hiccupping, abdominal pain and stomach ache.

7 照海 (Zhàohǎi) KI 6 Shining Sea 八脉交会穴通阴跷 Confluence points of the yin motility vessel

Location: On the medial side of the foot, in the depression inferior to the tip of the medial malleolus.

Acupuncture: Insert the needle perpendicularly to a depth of 0.5–0.8 cun and stimulate until there is a sore, numb sensation in the local area spreading in the ankle.

Moxibustion: Apply 3–5 moxa cones or hold a moxa stick above the point for 5–10 minutes.

Functions:

- Nourishes kidney and clears deficient heat
- Regulates yin motility vessel
- Relieves sore throat and calms the spirit
- Regulates the lower heater

Indications: Insomnia, manic psychosis, epilepsy, stroke and unconsciousness. Headache. Sore throat. Irregular menstruation, dysmenorrhea, morbid leucorrhea and mastitis. Frequent urination and enuresis. Constipation. Deafness. Dizziness. Dyspnea.

8 足临泣 (Zúlínqì) GB 41 Foot Supervising Tears 八脉交会穴通带脉 Confluence point of the belt vessel

Location: On the lateral aspect of the dorsum of the foot, posterior to the 4th metatarsophalangeal joint, in the depression on the lateral aspect of the tendon of the muscle extensor digit minimi of the foot.

Acupuncture:

1. Insert the needle perpendicularly to a depth of 0.5–0.8 cun and stimulate until there is a sore, numb sensation in the local area spreading to the toe.

2. Prick with a three-edged needle to bleed.

Moxibustion: Apply 3–5 moxa cones or needle-warming moxibustion or, alternatively, hold a moxa stick above the point for 5–10 minutes.

Functions:

- Spreads liver qi
- Pacifies wind and clears fire
- Clears the head and benefits the eyes

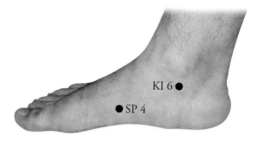

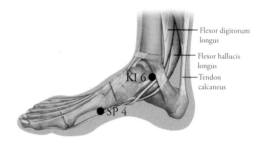

Flexor digitorum longus

Flexor hallucis longus

Tendon calcaneus

FIGURE 9.3

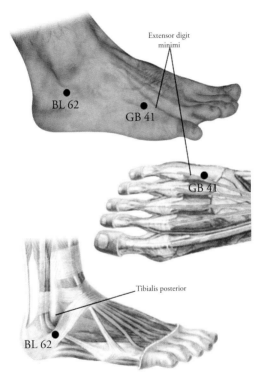

Extensor digit
minimi

BL 62

GB 41

GB 41

Tibialis posterior

BL 62

FIGURE 9.4